An Introduction to

Heat & Cold as Therapy

By **Laurel Fowlie** RMT, BA, MEd

 Curties-Overzet Publications

Many thanks to:

1. For the image on page 12: © Gunther von Hagens, Institute for Plastination, Heidelberg, Germany (www.bodyworlds.com)
2. For their Liquid Library stock photo images: © 2006 Inmagine JupiterImages Corporation
3. For permission to use their photographic images: Diane Deinstadt, Chiara Grisanzio, Jim Petersen, Winnie Wong, Jun Xiao

An Introduction to Heat & Cold as Therapy
Laurel Fowlie, RMT, BA, MEd
© Copyright 2006
Reprint 2015
To order copies, please contact:
Curties-Overzet Publications
330 Dupont Street, Suite 400
Toronto, Ontario
Canada M5R 1V9
Toll Free Phone: 1-888-649-5411
Fax: 416-923-8116
Website: www.curties-overzet.com
Email: info@curties-overzet.com

ISBN 978-0-9685256-5-4

Printed and bound in Canada by Thistle Printing Limited

Acknowledgements

For Joan

I would like to express my most enormous thanks to my parents and brother, Mary, George, and Wilson, for their endless support and encouragement, in this and all my endeavours.

I must say a huge thank you to my publisher, Debra Curties, for her advice, experience, and unending patience. Many thanks to the text readers: Cathy Fournier, Margaret Rockliffe, Peter Becker, and Sabine von Boetticher, who provided excellent comments and suggestions, and to the other knowledgeable people, including my colleagues Nadine Currie-Jackson and Candace Gerrior at the Atlantic College of Therapeutic Massage in Fredericton, who read the unfinished copy and offered valuable feedback. Also, my heartfelt appreciation goes to Bev Ransom for her illustrations and designs, to photographer Ellen Prose, and to proofreader Patsy Cunningham.

Shelley, Eileen, Raz, and André were all there when my knowledge of temperature therapy began back in Hamilton, and I couldn't have done it without them. I must express a big thank you to Carrie, Shampa, and Michelle who were all key in my becoming the instructor I am today. And thank you to Pete S., who demonstrated so well the importance of caution with contrast foot baths!

And, of course, a very special acknowledgement of Alisa who was there at the inception of the idea, and throughout the entire project with endless faith and encouragement.

Table of Contents

The word 'spa' is an acronym for 'salus per aquam', which is Latin for 'health from water.'

...

"We forget that the water cycle and the life cycle are one."

Jacques Cousteau

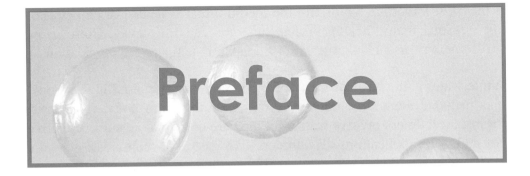

Preface

Hydrotherapy or Temperature Therapy?

The therapeutic use of hot and cold has traditionally been referred to as *hydrotherapy* because so many of the applications employed have been water-based – *hydro* means 'water'. Water is indeed an effective choice for such treatments. It can be used in any of its three forms: gas (steam), liquid (water), and solid (ice), and has been employed in healing for centuries because it is accessible, affordable, and has few adverse effects when used properly.

The human body is made of about 70% water, so water treatments work synergistically with the natural healing mechanisms of our bodies. The body's cells reside in watery fluids through which are transported the many elements they need for healthy function, such as nutrients, hormones, and substances for repair. Because the body and its activities are so fluid-based, water applications complement the natural functioning of the body.

It is essential to understand, however, that water is merely the medium through which the true therapeutic application, *temperature*, is applied. The therapeutic value of the treatments used in clinical practice (and in home care) comes from the temperature employed to achieve their effects. The *difference in temperature* between the source of the heat or cold and the part of the body to which it is being applied is what creates the therapeutic outcome. The application's temperature *in relation to the body's temperature* is the most important factor, not the medium that is heated or chilled. For this reason, many health professions are moving away from using 'hydrotherapy' as a blanket term for therapeutic temperature applications.

While water is the basis of many of the treatments discussed in this book, it is just one method of delivering temperature to the body. Gel packs, for instance, do not involve water, yet they are commonly used as effective hot and cold applications. Treatments like castor oil compresses do not employ water so it isn't accurate to call them hydrotherapy. Recently stones have become a popular therapeutic medium. For the sake of accuracy, then, the term *hydrotherapy* will only be used in this book when referring to a water-based treatment. We will refer to *thermotherapy* (*thermo*=heat) as the term for the therapeutic use of heat, and *cryotherapy* (*cryo*=cold) for the treatment of conditions with cold. The general term employed in this text to describe the use of heat and cold as treatment modalities is *temperature therapy*.

Temperature therapy has stood the test of time and continues to have an important place in a diverse range of health care disciplines. This textbook will start you along the path to understanding how it works and how to employ it safely and effectively in your clinical work.

try this:
Put one hand in hot water and the other hand in cold water. Then put both hands in warm water and note the difference in the feeling in each hand: the effects of temperature are relative.

Dr. Simon Baruch (1840-1921) of Poland taught his medical students that water has a place in *Materia Medica*, stating that "of all remedial agents in use since the dawn of medicine, water is the only one that has survived all the vicissitudes of doctrinal change."

Chapter One

Core Concepts

Learning Objectives

After learning the contents of this chapter, the reader should be able to:

- **define the main factor essential for temperature therapy to be effective**

- **demonstrate an understanding of the methods of heat transfer**

- **describe the thermal properties of water**

- **explain 'reaction'**

- **show an understanding of body temperature and its regulation**

- **demonstrate the complementary nature of temperature therapy and manual therapy**

- **explain the theory of local, systemic, and reflex effects of temperature therapy**

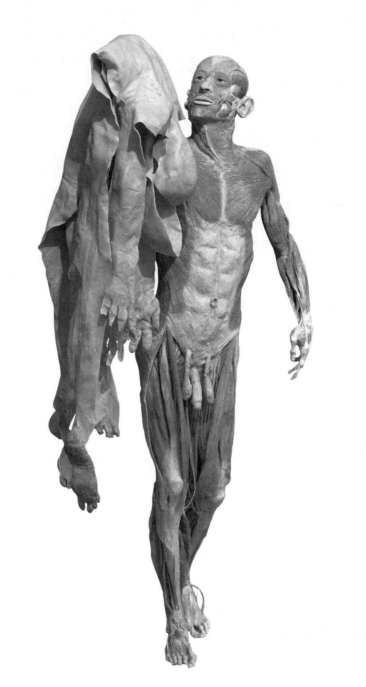

Figure 1.1: The skin is the body's largest organ.

Chapter 1: Core Concepts

Using temperature effectively depends on being able to intentionally mimic the natural influences that heat and cold have on the body. In order to use thermotherapy and cryotherapy properly, we must understand what their effects are and why. This includes having an awareness of the properties of skin and a basic understanding of the body's temperature regulation processes.

Equally important is the understanding of how heat is transferred between substances, including the role of water, which is the most commonly used therapeutic medium. This chapter introduces some elementary concepts about the body and its reactions to temperature.

Properties of the Skin

The skin is the body's access organ for temperature therapy. It is actually the body's largest organ, making up about 16% of the total body weight. On a typical adult, the skin covers about 2 m² (22 ft²). Averaging 1-2 mm (0.04-0.08"), the thickness of the skin varies from 0.5-4.0 mm (0.02-0.2").

The skin is structured into layers. The thinner, superficial layers of skin comprise the *epidermis*. The deeper section is the *dermis*, and the layer deep to the dermis is the *hypodermis*, or *subcutaneous (sub-Q)* layer.

• Epidermis

The more superficial epidermal layers contain cells that have completed their functions and have undergone scheduled death (*apoptosis*). The skin as we can see it, then, is comprised only of dead cells. The deeper layers of the epidermis have live, active cells which perform tasks that form and protect the skin.

• Dermis

The dermis contains proteins that give the skin its structure and pliability. *Collagen* is a very strong fibre that provides form and strength, and *elastin* gives skin its elasticity. Also found in the dermis are blood capillaries, nerve

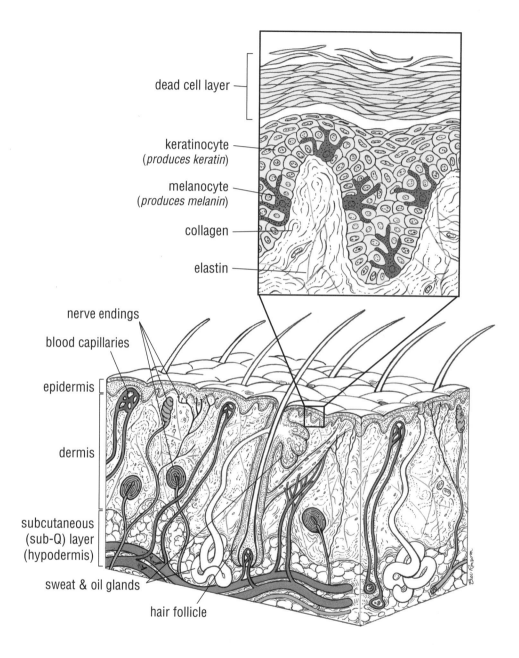

dead cell layer

keratinocyte
(*produces keratin*)

melanocyte
(*produces melanin*)

collagen

elastin

nerve endings

blood capillaries

epidermis

dermis

subcutaneous
(sub-Q) layer
(hypodermis)

sweat & oil glands

hair follicle

Figure 1.2: The structure of the skin.

endings (receptors), sweat and oil glands, and hair follicles. The nerve receptors in the dermis are the vehicles for providing sensation: touch, pressure, vibration, tickle, itch, pain, warmth, and cold.

• Subcutaneous Layer (Hypodermis)

The subcutaneous layer sits directly below the skin and contains blood vessels that supply the skin's capillary network, nerve fibres that conduct messages from the skin's receptors, and fat.

Skin Functions

Although we may tend to take our skin for granted, it plays some very important roles:

1. *Protection:* Skin performs a variety of protective tasks. It acts as a barrier to foreign substances, functioning as the body's first line of defence – bacteria, viruses, and fungi must have a port of entry in order to pass into the body. *Melanin* provides the brown pigment of the skin, which protects us from the sun's ultraviolet (UV) rays. *Keratin* toughens the skin and makes it durable. A fatty, or *lipid*, substance in the skin waterproofs it, keeping fluid in that is supposed to be inside the body and keeping fluid out that is supposed to stay outside. Skin can also reinforce itself protectively – continuous friction will cause the skin to develop a callus, which is a thickening that protects the underlying, more fragile structures.

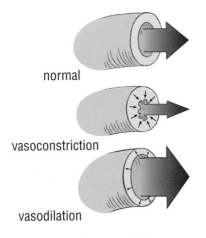

normal

vasoconstriction

vasodilation

Figure 1.3.

2. *Thermoregulation:* At rest, the dermis contains 8-10% of the body's blood flow, so the skin acts as a blood reservoir. This function of the skin is important to understand because of the key vascular effects of temperature therapy. Subcutaneous blood vessels change in diameter in response to heat and cold. They open up (*dilate*) in

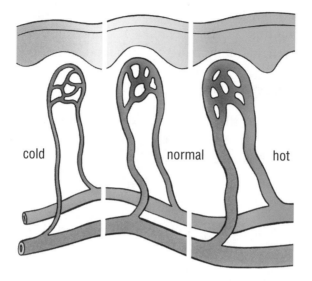

Figure 1.4: Cold on the skin's surface causes vasoconstriction of superficial capillaries, while heat results in vasodilation.

response to heat, filling capillaries that bring more blood flow to the body surface – in this way heat contained in the blood is allowed to escape. In reaction to cold, the blood vessels narrow (*constrict*), reducing the blood flow to the surface and promoting heat conservation in the body. Temperature applications can reproduce these natural responses to heat and cold for therapeutic purposes.

As well, sweat glands secrete water and waste products (*perspiration*). As perspiration evaporates from the skin surface heat leaves the body, so sweating is important in temperature regulation.

3. *Excretion:* Skin excretes salts, carbon dioxide, ammonia, and urea (a waste product produced by the kidneys during the production of urine). While it is not a primary organ of elimination, if the skin is healthy its elimination role helps reduce demand on other organs that act as toxin filters or eliminators (the kidneys, intestines, liver, lungs, and spleen). Used daily, temperature therapy can increase the efficiency of elimination and strengthen the body's general immunity.

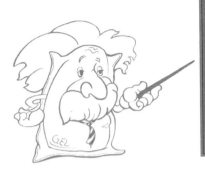

remember this:
The organs of filtration and elimination are S.K.I.L.L.S. :
Skin
Kidneys
Intestines
Liver
Lungs
Spleen

4. *Absorption:* Skin is also important for absorption, which is the movement of materials (good and bad) from outside the body into body cells. The role of absorption is significant therapeutically when additives are used in water. It is important to know the effects of any additives, such as oils or salts, that are used to enhance temperature therapy applications.

try this…
Put a couple of peeled cloves of garlic in your sock next to your skin. Monitor how long it takes for your breath to smell like garlic. See how well the skin absorbs substances into the body?

Reaction

In physiological terms, *reaction* refers to the body's healthy response to stress. Within reasonable parameters, it will respond to stressors by initiating *strengthening reactions* that increase the speed and efficiency of its feedback responses. Over time this enables the body to successfully withstand stronger and more frequent stressors. A feedback cycle is a primary means of adjusting to discomforts; it reflects changes in body function to adapt to a stimulus. For example, exercise causes changes in structures like skeletal muscle and the heart to increase the person's tolerance of exertion.

While stress can strengthen the body and its responses to stimuli, too much stress overwhelms defence mechanisms and leads to tissue damage. Temperature therapy can be seen as a form of strengthening stressor, but because of this potential for injury, it is important to be aware of contraindications to heat or cold. There are times when such applications are ill-advised or in need of modification. As well, hot and cold treatments can result in incomplete or negative reactions. Contraindications and negative reactions are discussed in later chapters.

Temperature therapy applications produce their effects through stimulating strengthening reactions of various types. To do so safely and effectively, they must stay within an appropriate temperature gradient. The body can withstand a temperature range of about 62°C (112°F). The skin's surface temperature is usually 28°-32°C (82°-90°F), but it can drop as far as 21°C (70°F) if uncovered at room temperature. The skin can tolerate a gel pack that is -5°C (23°F), and a paraffin wax treatment of 57°C (135°F).

Temperature Regulation

The body has narrow parameters within which its functions work properly. For example, when their temperature rises or drops too much, body systems are unable to function normally. Unless protective mechanisms are activated, death of the tissue, and of the individual, can occur. The *core temperature* is the temperature in structures that lie deep in the body, and is considered to be healthy at 37°C (98.6°F). The *shell temperature* is the temperature near the body's surface and is generally 1-6°C cooler than the core.

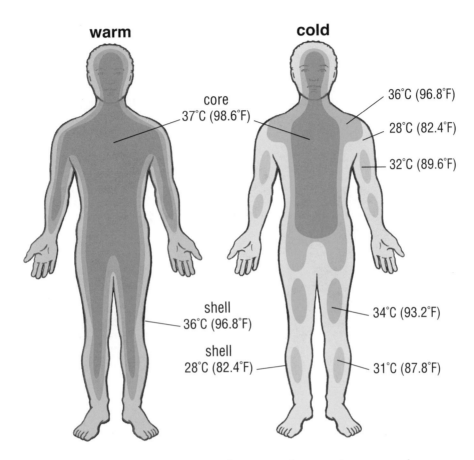

warm   cold

core
37°C (98.6°F)   36°C (96.8°F)

28°C (82.4°F)

32°C (89.6°F)

shell
36°C (96.8°F)   34°C (93.2°F)

shell
28°C (82.4°F)   31°C (87.8°F)

Figure 1.5: Shell temperature and core temperature.

Consider when your hands become very cold and fine activities such as writing seem impossible. An analogous effect occurs when the body's internal systems are affected by an excessive temperature change (hot or cold) and can no longer work properly. Because of this sensitivity, there are mechanisms in place that constantly regulate and adjust tissue temperature.

Keeping body functions constantly re-adjusting back to normal values involves a number of regulatory mechanisms. *Homeostasis* is the term used to represent the effects of all of the body's feedback cycles in maintaining healthy parameters. The hypothalamus, located in the brain, is important to homeostasis as the central nervous system's temperature regulator.

• The Role of the Hypothalamus in Temperature Regulation

Acting like a thermostat, the hypothalamus promotes heat conserving activities when the body is cold and heat losing activities when it is hot. It receives signals that keep it apprised of the temperature in the various body parts, and also monitors the temperature of the blood that passes through the hypothalamus itself.

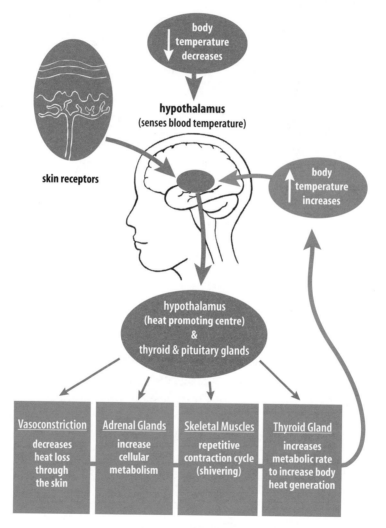

Figure 1.6a: Heat conserving activities.

1. *Heat Conserving Activities*: When blood that is cooled at the surface returns to the circulation deeper in the body, it stimulates heat conserving mechanisms initiated by the hypothalamus. Some activities that conserve body heat are shivering, goose bumps, and re-allocation of blood from the extremities to the body core. Shivering generates heat, as any body movement does. Goose bumps (*piloerection*) cause the body's hairs to stand erect and

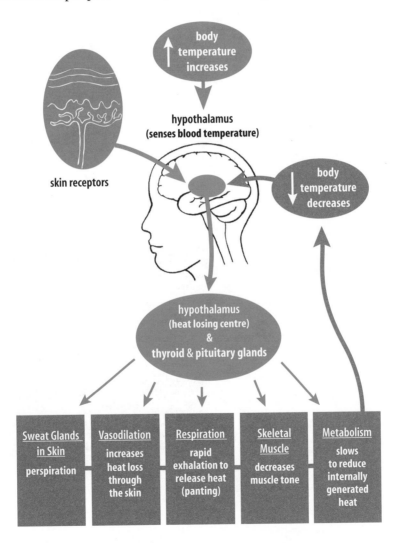

Figure 1.6b: Heat losing activities.

create an insulating layer of hair that traps air by the skin. Unfortunately, people no longer have thick coats of hair so this type of insulation is not as effective as it once was! Diverting blood to the inner part of the body helps keep the more important core temperature as warm as possible to protect proper functioning of the internal organs. A cold application, then, results in constriction of blood vessels (*vasoconstriction*) near the skin surface, directing blood flow toward the inner parts of the body.

2.   *Heat Losing Activities*: Perspiration, increased breathing rate, and dilation of the blood vessels near the skin surface are some of the ways in which the body strives to lose heat, again initiated by the hypothalamus. Perspiration is generally removed by evaporation, an action that results in cooling at the body surface. (Perspiration that drips off the body does not have the same cooling effect as perspiration that evaporates.) Rapid breathing allows the escape of heat via warm breath. The dilation of blood vessels (*vasodilation*) near the exterior of the body brings warm blood to the surface where the heat can escape into the surrounding air.

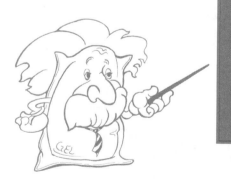

The hypothalamus receives signals that keep it apprised of the temperature in the various body parts, and also monitors the temperature of the blood that passes through the hypothalamus itself.

temperature regulation

- when the body is cold, heat conserving activities are initiated
- when the body is hot, heat losing activities are initiated

temp	activity	effect
cold	vasoconstriction	reduces heat loss via blood at the body's surface
	shivering	generates heat due to the movement
	goose bumps	hair creates an insulating layer which conserves heat at the surface of the skin
hot	vasodilation	increases heat loss via blood at the body's surface
	perspiring	evaporating perspiration cools the body's surface
	↑ breathing rate	heat escapes via the warm breath

Properties of Water

The body can be heated or cooled so effectively when water is the medium used because of water's thermal properties, namely *specific heat* and *thermal conductivity*:

- *Specific heat* is the capacity of a substance to *store* heat. Water can store four times more heat than air and twice as much as a paraffin wax mixture. That means that paraffin wax has about 50% less heat energy than water that is at the same temperature.

- *Thermal conductivity* is the capacity of a substance to *conduct* heat to other substances or materials. The higher the conductivity of a material, the better that material transfers heat. The thermal conductivity of solids is about 100 times that of liquids, which have about 100 times more conductivity than gases. This difference in conductivity explains why, for instance, moist hot towels provide a more effective treatment than dry ones.

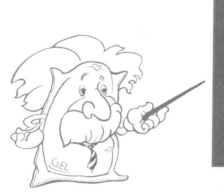

Specific heat is the capacity of a substance to store heat; thermal conductivity is the capacity of a substance to transfer heat to other substances.

In addition to its thermal properties, water can also be effective as a therapeutic medium because of mechanical and chemical effects. The term *mechanical effects* refers to the stimulation that results from water striking the body, such as with a shower or water jets. *Chemical effects* are present when substances such as salts or oils are added to the water and the resulting mixture is used on the body.

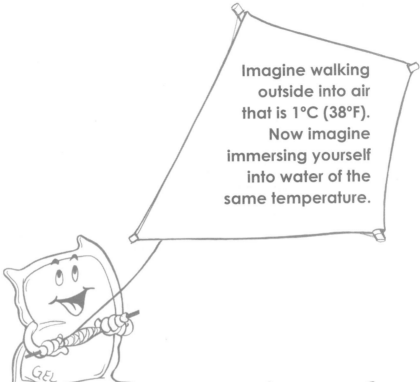

Imagine walking outside into air that is 1°C (38°F). Now imagine immersing yourself into water of the same temperature.

GEL

Figure 1.7:
Even though these towels are heated to the same temperature, the moist one will feel hotter. This is because water is an excellent temperature conductor.

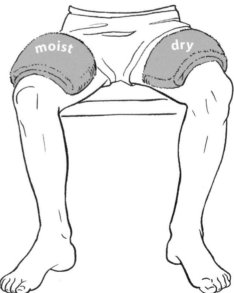

moist   dry

Transfer of Heat

Heat transfer is an exchange of energy between two materials that occurs in relation to the temperature difference between the two materials. A heat treatment will have a different effect on a warmed body part than on the same area after it has been chilled. *Cold is defined as the relative absence of heat*. Rather than adding cold to a body part, then, cold applications remove heat from it.

Heat transfer (heating and cooling body tissues) occurs by five methods. Our treatments transfer temperature using one or more of these methods.

Rather than adding cold to a body part, cryotherapy removes heat from it.

They are:

- conduction

- convection

- evaporation

- radiation

- conversion

Conduction is the exchange of heat between two surfaces that are in direct contact with each other. For example, an electric heating pad lying on the body transmits heat to the tissue by conduction.

Convection is the result of movement of a heated gas or liquid between surfaces at different temperatures. For instance, when the hot air of a sauna touches the body's cooler skin, the body becomes warmed.

Evaporation is the conversion of a liquid to a vapour. Each millilitre of evaporated water takes heat with it as it evaporates, as in perspiration. Note that perspiration that drips off the body rather than evaporates does not remove much heat.

Radiation is the transfer of heat between objects via infrared rays. Radiation requires no direct contact between the objects. The heat that the body absorbs when in sunshine is an example of radiation.

Conversion involves no externally applied heat, but uses energy coursing through a substance to heat it. Ultrasound is an example of conversion.

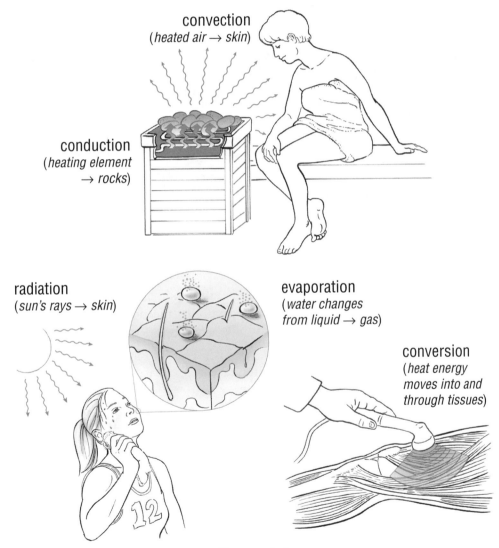

Figure 1.8.

means of heat exchange

means	how it works	example
conduction	surfaces in contact	hot pack
convection	heated gas/liquid moving between areas	steam treatments
evaporation	conversion of liquid to vapour	perspiration
radiation	infrared rays	sunshine
conversion	energy through the substance	ultrasound

Manual Therapies

Because using heat and cold for therapy is typically gentle and natural, such applications are complementary to other healing modalities. Thermotherapy and cryotherapy have similar effects on many of the body systems as, for example, massage. Heat treatments and deep massage using petrissage strokes, for instance, both decrease muscle tone. Conversely, stimulating techniques such as tapotement can increase muscle tone, creating similar effects as a cold treatment. Sometimes it is a matter of choosing the modality best suited to achieve the desired effect in the individual client's body.

Many practitioners combine temperature therapies with manual treatment to achieve enhanced effects, for example, by applying thermotherapy over a muscle group before a massage treatment. Sometimes temperature therapy is used to mitigate the effects of manual treatment, as with the use of aggressive techniques like frictioning. Since frictioning can generate an inflammatory response in the treated tissues, cold therapy (e.g., ice massage) is usually partnered with the manual treatment to control the results.

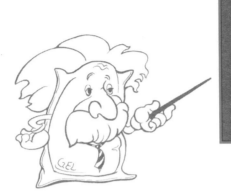

Many therapists combine temperature therapy modalities with manual treatment to achieve enhanced effects.

Temperature therapy and manual therapies generally have fewer adverse effects than medications that could be prescribed for the same condition. As well, because of the accessibility of temperature therapy, such treatments can actively involve an individual in her or his own care.

In addition to the ways clients benefit, practitioners of manual therapies can make excellent use of temperature therapy in their own self care. Just as an example, warm water on the hands before performing a treatment and cold water afterward can promote good perfusion and drainage to optimize function. Temperature therapy can also play an important role in injury prevention and maintenance of occupationally overused body areas.

Effects of Temperature Therapy Applications

• Local Effects

In many instances, temperature therapies are applied as *local* treatments; that is, to a specific body area or body part. Their results are intentionally local, ensuing from the effects of increasing or decreasing blood flow, altering local immune responses, and improving pliability of the tissue.

• Reflex Effects

The primary means by which hot and cold treatments affect the internal organs is through *reflex effects*, since their temperature isn't actually changed by the applications. In the context of temperature therapy, a reflex is a reaction in response to a stimulus that is applied to the periphery of the body but enacted in a deeper structure through the mediation of the central nervous system (CNS). These are programmed reflex responses to adapt to the CNS's perception of the intent of the stimulus, for example to increase/decrease glandular activity, alter blood flow into the structure, and so on.

These reflex patterns can be used therapeutically to stimulate the body surface and produce desired effects in deeper structures, since treating the skin in a reflex area can address the related organ. Often the section of skin that overlies an organ is the reflex area for that organ; however, some reflex areas are more distant, as you can see in Figure 1.10.

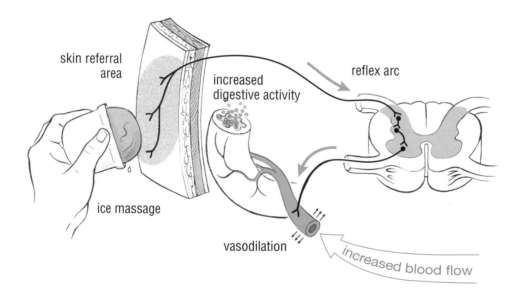

Figure 1.9: Cryotherapy applied to the reflex zone on the abdomen surface can promote increased digestive activity.

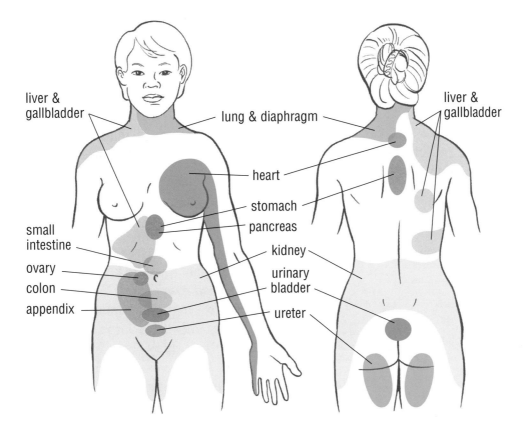

liver &
gallbladder

lung & diaphragm

liver &
gallbladder

heart

stomach

pancreas

small
intestine

ovary

colon

appendix

kidney

urinary
bladder

ureter

Figure 1.10: Visceral reflex referral zones on the skin surface.

Reflex effects are classified into three categories based on their functions:

- vasomotor

- visceromotor

- glandular

Vasomotor effects are the ways a stimulus affects the smooth muscle of the blood vessels supplying a tissue, leading to constriction or dilation of the vessels.

Visceromotor effects are the effects that temperature change has on the smooth muscle tissue of the viscera. The smooth muscle is what causes movement within an organ.

Glandular effects are the effects temperature therapy can have on glandular secretions (e.g., mucus, enzymes, hormones).

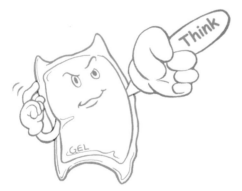

An important reflex to keep in mind is the *arterial trunk reflex*. Whatever the influence a temperature therapy treatment has on a large artery, the same effect may be conveyed to smaller blood vessels branching off the primary artery. In conditions where heat is contraindicated, for instance, it is important to be aware of this type of reflex: if you want to apply heat to the thigh, consider the needs of the lower leg as well, because the lower leg's vessels are continuous with those in the upper leg.

• Systemic Effects

Temperature therapies can be applied to the whole body, creating significant additional *systemic effects*. With a bath or a whirlpool, for example, the pressure exerted on body tissues and cavities by the water in which the person is immersed creates changes beyond those caused by the temperature itself. The pressure of the water increases venous pressure, increasing blood flow back to the heart. With a hot application, there is also an increase in the heart rate; the heart rate will slow down if the treatment is cold.

Increased venous return to the heart also causes a larger volume of blood to be pushed into the thorax, reducing the amount of space the lungs have available to fill with air. Breathing increases in difficulty with full body treatments, so individuals being treated must be monitored, particularly if they have a history of respiratory difficulties.

Full body heat treatments also cause an overall increase in blood flow to the skin, subcutaneous tissues, and superficial muscles.

As we proceed to take a more detailed look at the effects of heat, cold and contrast applications in the next three chapters, more information will be added to refine our understanding of how the effects of temperature therapies can be directed to achieve specific therapeutic goals.

Sebastian Kneipp (1821-1897) of Germany had pulmonary tuberculosis in the 1840s, at a time when the disease was usually fatal. He read a hydrotherapy book, On the Healing Virtues of Cold Water, Inwardly and Outwardly Applied, as Proved by Experience *from the 1730s by a Dr. Hahn, and decided to try some techniques. Kneipp immersed himself several times a week in the freezing Danube River, which appeared to bolster his immune system because his TB went into remission. He published* My Water Cure *in 1866, a book which recommended bathing in and drinking cold water, going to bed and rising early, and taking long walks barefoot in the grass. He believed that if a person were diseased, water would "dissolve, remove, and strengthen." He was once arraigned for quackery, of which he was eventually acquitted.*

Chapter Two

Physiological Effects of Cold

Learning Objectives

After learning the contents of this chapter, the reader should be able to:

- define retrostasis

- explain the hunting response and active derivation

- demonstrate an understanding of the first stage of the inflammatory response and how cold addresses the effects of acute inflammation

- list the five cardinal signs and symptoms of inflammation

- explain hypoxia

- define the countercurrent heat exchange of blood vessels

- demonstrate an understanding of the factors that influence the effects of cold

- identify the direct and reflex effects of cold

- identify common indications for the use of cryotherapy

- show understanding of cautions related to the use of cold

hypothermic comas for central nervous system injuries

Doctors at the Foothills Hospital in Calgary, Alberta, and at Memorial Hermann Hospital in Houston, Texas, are studying the effects of inducing a hypothermic coma for the treatment of acquired brain and spinal cord injuries.

The procedure involves lowering the body temperature to 34°C/93.2°F (36°-38°C/96.8°-100.4°F is normal). Ideally, this should be done within 90-120 minutes of the injury. The body, which goes into hibernation mode, slows its functions so blood-borne oxygen is conserved and can be concentrated to heal the injured nervous tissue. Bleeding and swelling are also greatly reduced.

The potential benefits of hypothermic coma were found because of a "laboratory accident." One of the doctors involved was supervising a drug test for central nervous system injuries induced in lab animals. The experimenters noticed that in the winter, when the temperature went down in the older building where the experiments were being held, control animals who did not receive the drug therapy treatment were still not showing signs of their injuries.

Doctors are currently running a human study which will involve 240 subjects.

http://www.ctv.ca/servlet/ArticleNews/story/CTVNews/20060303/WFIVE_on_ice_060303

Chapter 2: Physiological Effects of Cold

What effects does cold have on the body? Most of the time the reaction is depressive, meaning that cold tends to slow down metabolic functions. The effects of cryotherapy may also be stimulating – this tends to occur if the application is brief or is used to achieve reflex effects.

Cold modalities work by extracting heat from the warmer skin. The greater the temperature difference between the application and the skin, the larger the drop in tissue temperature. Cooling of the body surface initiates responses that underpin the effects of cold: retrostasis, heat conservation, and the hunting response.

Retrostasis and Heat Conservation

When a tissue requires blood or fluid for any reason, that fluid will be drawn from an area of congestion first. Likewise, if the heat of warm blood is needed in a body part, it will be shunted in from other body parts that have excess blood. *Retrostasis*, the result of blood vessel constriction in the skin and subcutaneous tissues, is the action of fluid being mobilized from the body surface into deeper tissues and internal organs. Cold applications utilize these reactions to move blood away from or into desired tissue zones.

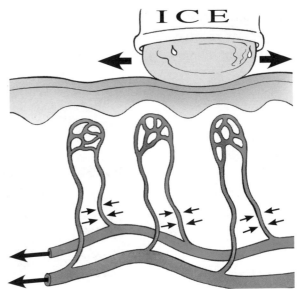

Figure 2.1:
Cryotherapy produces vasoconstriction in superficial capillaries, keeping blood moving toward deeper tissues.

When the body constricts the superficial blood vessels in response to cold, it is also activating a protective heat-conserving mechanism to minimize heat loss through the skin. Vasoconstriction at the body surface limits the amount of blood circulating through the skin and subcutaneous tissues, restricting the amount of heat that can be released. This vasoconstriction complements the cold-induced retrostasis because it aids blood flow into the deeper tissues and resists flow toward the skin surface.

Hunting Response

Another event that happens in response to an application of cold is the *hunting response*. The hunting response occurs when the temperature in a tissue is reduced for 12-15 minutes or more, or when it is brought below 10°C (50°F). Under such conditions a cold-induced vasodilation follows the initial vasoconstriction. This vasodilation is referred to as *derivation*, which is the drawing of fluid from its main pathway, away from a higher volume area toward the chilled tissue. What ensues are cyclic periods of vasodilation and vasoconstriction, and therefore increased and decreased temperature in the cool region. During these cycles, however, the tissue does not return to the pre-treatment temperature.

The hunting response is an attempt by the body to ensure that peripheral body parts receive sufficient blood when exposed to cold so that they can resist tissue damage (i.e., frostbite). The magnitude and frequency of the

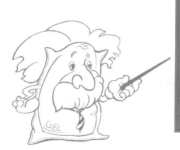

The hunting response occurs when the temperature in a tissue is reduced for 12-15 minutes or more, or when it is brought below 10°C (50°F), causing cyclic periods of vasodilation and vasoconstriction to help the tissue resist cold-induced damage.

hunting response is in direct relationship to the person's core body temperature. This protective mechanism is only useful if the individual has a relatively warm core temperature while subjected to cold, so may not prevent tissue damage when the entire body is exposed to severe cold. The vasodilation that occurs in the hunting response is active derivation, meaning that the body must expend energy in order for the derivation to occur.

Inflammation and Cryotherapy

One of the main uses of cold applications is the management of inflammation, especially in the acute stage. The *inflammatory response* is the body's non-specific reaction to damage, meaning that inflammation occurs regardless of the type of damaging stimulus. The primary functions of inflammation are to dispose of foreign entities (e.g., bacteria) at the site of injury, to prevent spread of those foreign entities beyond the site, and to prepare the injured tissues for repair.

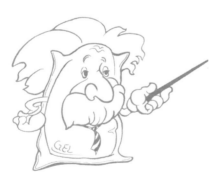

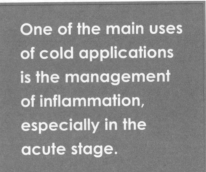

One of the main uses of cold applications is the management of inflammation, especially in the acute stage.

A key event in inflammation, important to the rationale for our use of cold treatments, is *vasodilation and increased permeability* of the blood vessels supplying the damaged tissue. When a blood vessel dilates the diameter of its *lumen* (inner cavity) increases, which allows a great deal more blood to flow through the tissue. This increase in blood flow facilitates two important things: first, the nutrients and cells that are needed for repair are able to get there faster; and second, waste products and fluid accumulation are more efficiently removed.

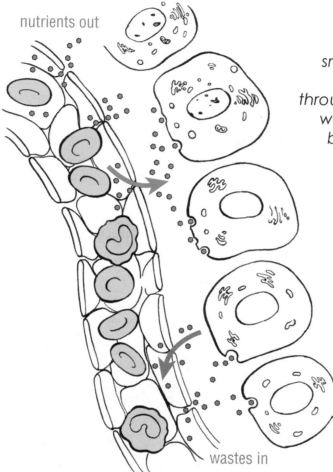

nutrients out

wastes in

Figure 2.2a:
Normal capillary
dynamics, where
small-sized nutrients
and wastes pass
through the capillary's
walls and the larger
blood cells do not.

The *permeability* of a vessel refers to how easily substances pass through the vessel's wall. Permeability relates mainly to capillaries, which are the tiny vessels in contact with their tissues' cells. It is through these capillaries that nutrients and metabolic wastes are exchanged between the tissue and the bloodstream. The more permeable a capillary becomes, the more material can pass through freely. The increase in capillary permeability that comes with the inflammatory process permits larger items that would not normally leave the blood to enter the tissues. In this way, the specific cells that help defend and repair the body can travel to the damaged tissue.

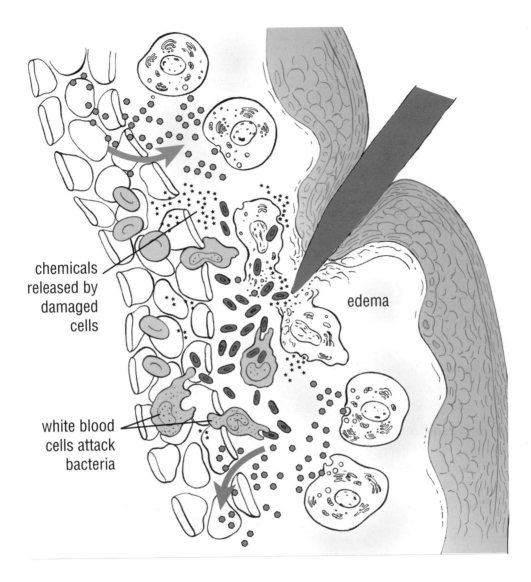

chemicals
released by
damaged
cells

edema

white blood
cells attack
bacteria

Figure 2.2b: Chemicals released by damaged cells enter the
bloodstream and activate pain and inflammation responses.
During inflammation greater capillary wall permeability
permits increased nutrient delivery and waste removal, as
well as passage of white blood cells and other elements
necessary for the immune response and for tissue repair.

Vasodilation and increased permeability in early inflammation contribute to what are called the cardinal signs of inflammation:

- *Redness* is the result of the large volume of blood that has entered the tissue and is called *hyperemia*. Depending on the person's skin colour, there will be obvious redness or pronounced darkening of the skin.

- *Heat* is due to the extra blood accumulation, plus the rise in the metabolic rate that occurs as part of the immune and healing processes. The hotter the body the faster chemical reactions occur, and the more metabolic activity is taking place, the more heat is generated. A cycle develops that sustains heat at the site for some time.

- *Swelling* (edema) results from the increase in capillary permeability, which allows not only nutrients and cells but also additional fluid to pass through the blood vessel wall into the interstitium (the spaces between the body cells).

- *Pain* is usually due to substances released by injured cells and perhaps from the release of chemicals from an invading agent. If nerves are damaged, this may add to the pain, as may pressure from the increased fluid volume on the injured and neighbouring structures.

- *Altered function* is caused by the pain and swelling, the injury itself, and the protective muscle guarding that almost inevitably occurs. In musculoskeletal structures this usually presents as reduced mobility.

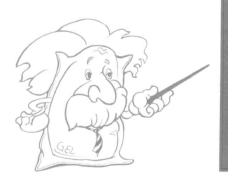

remember this:
There are 5 characteristic signs and symptoms of inflammation (S.H.A.R.P.):
Swelling
Heat
Altered Function
Redness
Pain

Stages of Inflammation

As the inflammatory response activates, progresses and subsides, the tissue is said to go through three stages: *acute*, *sub-acute*, and *chronic*. Acute inflammation is the swelling stage and manifests with the cardinal signs listed above.

Sub-acute inflammation is the regenerating stage in which healing and repair are initiated. Edema and hyperemia begin to diminish and any bruising starts to change colour and resolve. Local range of motion begins to increase, but there may continue to be pain, and the tissue remains fragile.

Chronic inflammation is the scar tissue and healing stage. In this phase there are few visible signs of inflammation at the site – perhaps some cool edema and point tenderness – and scar tissue becomes increasingly effective in securing the injured tissue. Reduced range of motion can persist because of local adhesions and/or muscle tension. Resolution of the injury brings the chronic stage of inflammation to a natural end; prolonged symptoms usually indicate that the tissues are not healing properly or the site has been re-injured, often due to premature activity.

Each stage of the inflammation process requires a different treatment approach. With respect to temperature therapy the general rule is: cold for acute, contrast for sub-acute, and heat for chronic. (Hot and contrast treatments will be discussed in upcoming chapters.) This rule is over-simplistic, since there are cases where these approaches can be varied or should be adapted, especially in the sub-acute and chronic stages. As a universal rule, however, 'cold for acute' is strongly adhered to. Heat should never be applied to acutely inflamed tissue.

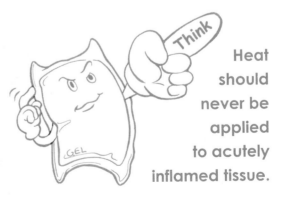

Think

Heat should never be applied to acutely inflamed tissue.

Why Cold is Effective

The body's inflammatory response is often excessive relative to the injury. Because of this, helping to control the intensity of inflammation reduces symptoms and potential complications. Cryotherapy helps minimize the degree of vasodilation that occurs – remember that a key effect of a cold application is superficial vasoconstriction. Another important benefit of vasoconstriction at an injury site is that blood loss (internal or external) is minimized by narrowing of the affected blood vessels. The more constricted a blood vessel is, the less blood can travel through and escape the body or pool at the site as bruising or a contusion.

Figure 2.3.

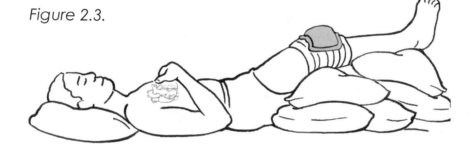

When placing cold on an acute injury, it is best to combine the cryotherapy with compression and elevation. Local pressure and elevation of the body part above the level of the pumping heart help to reduce blood loss and to control accumulation of fluid (edema) around the injury.

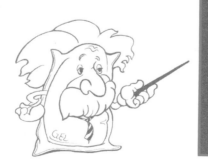

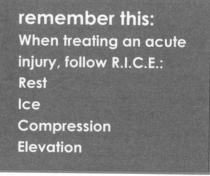

remember this:
When treating an acute injury, follow R.I.C.E.:
Rest
Ice
Compression
Elevation

The early closing of a wound is created by soft granulation tissue. *Fibroblasts*, the cells that lay down scar tissue, travel to the site to create a sturdier, permanent resolution. While scar tissue is essential to the healing process it can also be overproduced. Scars are not made of functional tissue, so they can impede efficient tissue performance. The vasoconstriction induced by cryotherapy prevents excessive fibroblast migration and activity, helping control the amount of scar tissue developed and therefore the amount of dysfunction it might cause.

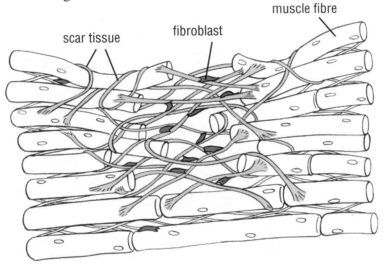

Figure 2.4: While scars unite and stabilize an injury site, they can also reduce tissue performance and be a source of irritation and pain.

The onset of acute inflammation can cause secondary hypoxic injury as a result of the effects of swelling or of accumulation of metabolic wastes. *Hypoxia* refers to inadequate oxygen supply and its damaging effect on cells. Cells in and around the damaged tissue can be further compromised by oxygen deprivation.

Inadequate oxygen delivery can be compounded if there is damage to the blood vessels that supply uninjured, peripheral cells in the affected tissue zone. The vasoconstriction and slower local metabolism that result from a cold application help reduce hypoxia. By reducing the metabolic rate, the cells' oxygen demand is minimized. The cells at and around the trauma site are then better equipped to cope with a temporary period of reduced oxygen availability.

In addition to helping control the physiological events of inflammation, an application of cold also relieves pain via the anaesthetic effect of numbing local nerve endings and elevating the individual's pain threshold.

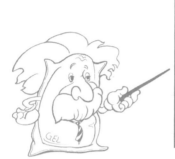

In addition to helping control the physiological events of inflammation, an application of cold also relieves pain by numbing nerve endings and raising the local pain threshold.

Ideally, cold should be applied immediately after trauma in order to reduce the extent of soft tissue damage from cell death and hemorrhage, and to decrease the inflammation. After the inflammation is well established, cryotherapy can still function as a painkiller and antispasmodic, but will have less effect on the inflammatory response. Once swelling has been minimized, the cold treatment should be discontinued so healing is not delayed by lengthy vasoconstriction. The best approach with acute injuries is usually to apply cold, remove for a period of time, then re-apply so that inflammation is controlled but local blood flow is kept adequate for transport of the necessary cells and nutrients, and metabolism is sufficient for the healing processes to get under way.

In addition to addressing inflammation, cold treatments are effective in helping manage fevers. Full body applications like cool washings are generally most helpful in reducing fever. Brief washings should be applied so as not to hinder perspiration, since perspiring is the body's natural way of lowering its temperature (heat-losing activity), and this mechanism should not be inhibited. Intermittent washings are best since they provide relief without over-treating – fever is an important part of the immune response.

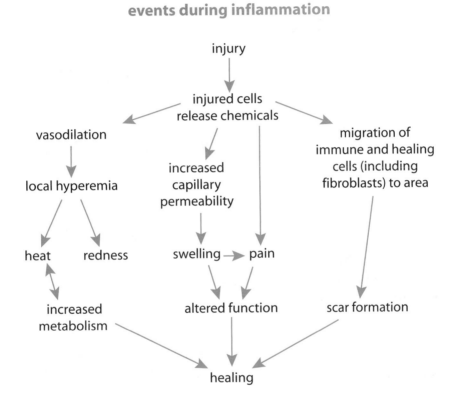

events during inflammation

Duration of Effects of Cold

Arterial blood (blood in the arteries) carries oxygenated, nutrient-rich blood from the heart to body tissues, while *venous* blood (blood in the veins) carries deoxygenated blood with waste products from body tissues back to the heart. As blood reaches the surface of the body, heat in the blood is released to the external environment. Normally, as warm arterial blood from the body's core travels to the peripheral tissues and passes by the cooler returning venous blood, there is a *countercurrent heat exchange*. That is to say, as the arterial and venous blood pass each other, the arterial blood warms the cooler venous blood, and the venous blood cools the warmer arterial blood.

The vasoconstriction caused by a cold application reduces the amount of warm blood entering a tissue area. The countercurrent heat exchange is reduced and the tissue will not re-warm as quickly as usual. Cold penetrates deeper into tissue than heat because the presence of cold related vasoconstriction reduces the arrival of fresh warm blood that can diminish the influence of the cold. The effects of cold also last longer than those of heat since a cooled area takes longer to return to resting temperature than warmed tissue because of the effects of cold on blood flow.

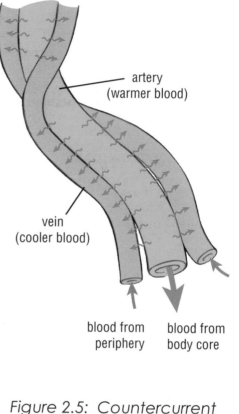

artery
(warmer blood)

vein
(cooler blood)

blood from periphery

blood from body core

Figure 2.5: Countercurrent heat exchange between warm arterial blood and cooler incoming venous blood.

As has already been mentioned, prolonged intermittent cryotherapy is superior to a single cold application. This type of treatment protocol sustains the desired effects of cold while minimizing potential negative effects. As well, the cold applications can be removed before activation of the hunting response takes place, thereby avoiding its vasodilation (derivation) effects.

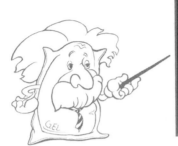

A longer protocol of intermittent cryotherapy is superior to a single cold application. This type of treatment protocol sustains the desired effects of cold while minimizing potential negative effects and avoiding the vasodilation of the hunting response.

Influences on Cold's Effects

The form of cold application used impacts the degree of cooling. A dynamic ice massage, in which ice is continuously moved over the target tissue, has greater results than, for instance, a static cold gel pack application which tends to become warmed by the body tissues.

The colder the application, the more intense the vasoconstriction. Extreme cold is more tolerable if the cold source is not kept continuously on the tissue; a mobile application accomplishes the desired results more efficiently. Percussive techniques coupled with cold make the cryotherapy more tolerable for an individual who dislikes cold applications. The percussion functions as a distraction to reduce the perception of cold intensity. Care must be taken with such techniques, however, because the numbing effects of the cryotherapy may decrease the perception of pain.

The physical characteristics of the individual receiving the treatment have a significant impact on its efficacy. The greater the temperature difference between the skin and the cooling source, the greater the resulting temperature change. Someone who is warm will experience greater effects than a person who is chilled.

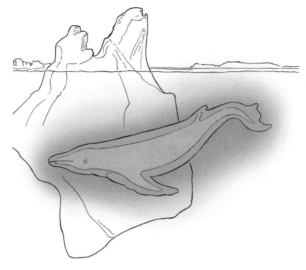

Figure 2.6:
Fat is a powerful temperature insulator. For example, even in frigid waters the temperature of the whale's warm-blooded body systems is maintained because of the insulating effects of a thick subcutaneous fat layer.

The amount of subcutaneous fatty (*adipose*) tissue the recipient has affects the rate of temperature reduction when cold is applied, and of re-warming when it is removed. The adipose is not the target tissue, and its additional thickness can reduce the effectiveness of the cold treatment in addressing its target. Fatty tissue is a poor conductor of temperature, acting as an insulator and impairing cold's ability to reach and affect the tissues below it. Similarly, structures with little or no adipose covering, like bony prominences, can be overchilled by prolonged cryotherapy.

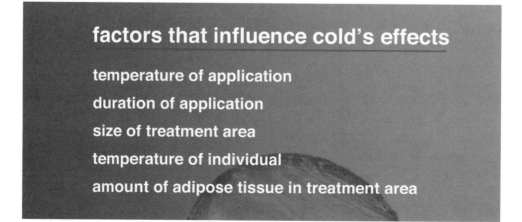

factors that influence cold's effects

temperature of application

duration of application

size of treatment area

temperature of individual

amount of adipose tissue in treatment area

Direct Effects of Cold

Cold, as previously mentioned, has depressive effects on tissue metabolism when the treatment is prolonged, while short applications are stimulating.

• Brief Cryotherapy Applications

Brief cold (<1 minute) is stimulating because of immediate vasoconstriction followed by a counteracting vasodilation response (active derivation). This activity of the blood vessels brings a fresh supply of oxygen and nutrients to the cells, optimizing their ability to perform their tasks.

• Longer Cryotherapy Applications

Cold applications of longer duration have sedative effects including slowing of metabolism in the treated tissues. They also cause shunting of blood away from the treated body surface area. These effects are central to the rationale for using cryotherapy in most cases.

In addition to reducing body temperature and metabolism, larger scale cryotherapy applications also decrease the heart and breathing rates. With slower metabolism comes diminished need for oxygen to be inhaled and pumped to the tissues, and a reduction in the amount of carbon dioxide and other waste that must be returned to the heart and lungs for removal from the body.

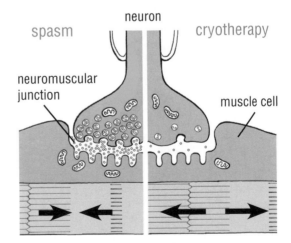

Most types of muscle spasms can be addressed with cold therapy. The cooler a muscle is, the slower the rate of firing of the nerve impulses that cause the muscle to contract. Neurons demonstrate less

Figure 2.7: Cold reduces transmission across the neuromuscular junction.

frequent conduction as they cool, and transmission becomes greatly reduced where the neuron meets the muscle cell (*neuromuscular junction*). There is a direct relationship between neuron temperature and frequency of impulses causing muscle fibre contraction.

Not only does cold reduce motor neuron impulse activity, it also decreases *muscle spindle* sensitivity. Muscle spindles are receptors found in skeletal muscles. Their function is to monitor stretch in the muscle and to initiate a countering reflex to prevent overstretch injury. Because these receptors are

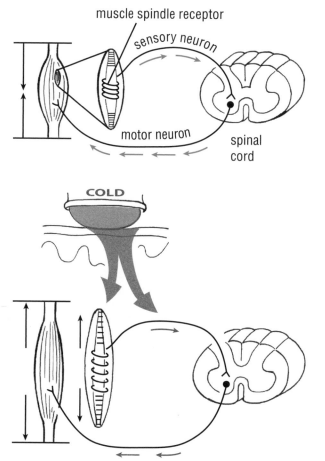

Figure 2.8a: When a muscle is tense or spasmed, small movements elicit strong muscle spindle responses that tend to prolong the spasm.

Figure 2.8b: Cooling the spindle receptor apparatus makes it less sensitive to stretch and helps release the muscle spasm.

responsible for inducing muscle contraction, their desensitization reduces muscle tension and therefore can help treat muscle spasm. It should be noted, however, that if the primary cause of a muscle spasm is ischemia (decreased oxygen supply), heat is usually a more appropriate treatment choice.

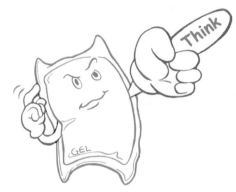

While cold helps reduce muscle spasm by slowing neuronal activity, if the primary cause of a spasm is ischemia heat is a more appropriate temperature therapy choice.

Joint pain and inflammation can often be decreased with cold. As cold compresses are applied, the temperature of the skin drops first, then of the subcutaneous soft tissue, then the intra-articular region (inside the joint). As little as five minutes of cold can reduce intra-articular temperature, helping relieve joint swelling and discomfort.

A less desirable result of longer cold applications is increased viscosity of the local tissue environment, which can lead to decreased plasticity and therefore resistance to motion, reduced dexterity, and slower reaction time. The downside for some individuals is that they may experience joint stiffness secondary to cryotherapy applications.

direct effects of cold

- **brief treatment**

area	effect
any	brief vasoconstriction followed by vasodilation; refreshes local blood supply and stimulates tissue performance

- **longer treatment**

area	effect
any	induces vasoconstriction and retrostasis, then vasodilation and active derivation
inflamed tissue	reduces inflammation and pain
metabolic rate	slows
respiratory system	sedates
cardiovascular system	sedates
abdomen	stimulates underlying viscera
kidneys	increases function
muscles	eases spasms
joints	decreases swelling; can increase stiffness

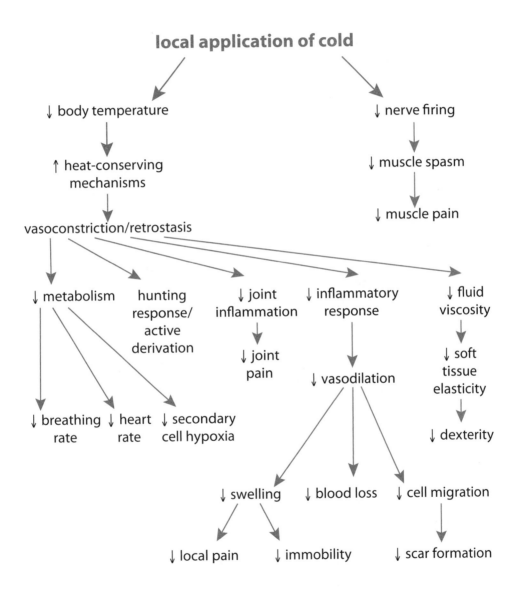

local application of cold

↓ body temperature

↓ nerve firing

↑ heat-conserving mechanisms

↓ muscle spasm

↓ muscle pain

vasoconstriction/retrostasis

↓ metabolism

hunting response/ active derivation

↓ joint inflammation

↓ inflammatory response

↓ fluid viscosity

↓ breathing rate

↓ heart rate

↓ secondary cell hypoxia

↓ joint pain

↓ vasodilation

↓ soft tissue elasticity

↓ dexterity

↓ swelling

↓ blood loss

↓ cell migration

↓ local pain

↓ immobility

↓ scar formation

Reflex Effects of Cold

Cryotherapy applications can have effects beyond the tissue area to which the cold is applied. While its effects on local tissue metabolism are generally depressive, cold can be used reflexively to stimulate activity in target organs. Despite the inability of the cold to actually reach the organs, these effects happen because of retrostasis. (See *Figure 1.10* in Chapter 1 for a reflex referral zone chart.) Reflex effects of cryotherapy can be produced with both brief and longer treatments.

• Brief Cryotherapy Applications

Brief cold (can include percussive touch) to the skin surface reflex area of an organ increases the organ's functional activity. On the chest, with friction or percussion, cold induces an immediate increase in the respiration rate, followed by slower, deeper breathing. Applied over the heart, brief cold results in an increased heart rate. A short cold treatment on the hands, face, and head stimulates the central nervous system to increase mental activity and alertness. Brief cold can also enhance digestion, urine production, elimination, respiration, pulse rate, immune functioning, and muscle tone via reflex effects.

• Longer Cryotherapy Applications

Prolonged cold to the nose and back of the neck causes contraction of blood vessels in the nasal mucosa, which can be very helpful with nosebleeds. An extended cold treatment on the abdomen increases blood flow to the intestines, making more blood available for nutrient absorption from the digestive organs. A prolonged treatment of cold over the heart reduces the heart rate. An extended cold application over the kidneys provides a fresh blood supply, enhancing their efficiency. A long cold treatment to the scalp contracts the blood vessels in the head, which can help relieve migraine headaches (providing the tissue temperature is increased gradually on removal of the cold to avoid headache rebound).

reflex effects of cold

brief treatment

area	effect
charted reflex area	stimulates the organ's activities
chest	temporarily $\uparrow$ the breathing rate
over heart	$\uparrow$ heart rate
hands, face, head	$\uparrow$ mental activity

longer treatment

area	effect
nose, back of neck	vasoconstriction in nasal mucosa
over heart	$\downarrow$ heart rate
scalp	vasoconstriction in head
kidneys	stimulates filtration function
abdomen	stimulates blood flow, motility and absorption in digestive organs

Indications for Cold Applications

There are many conditions for which cold is generally indicated. It is important to take a thorough case history and to do an appropriate assessment in order to determine any cautions or contraindications in the individual case, but the following are conditions for which cold is typically helpful:

- acute sprains and strains

- acute soft tissue trauma in general, including contusions

- inflammation

- edema

- muscular pain

- muscle guarding, muscle spasm (except when ischemia is the primary cause)

- acute tendonitis

- acute bursitis

- fractures

- post-surgical conditions

- headaches, migraines

- hemorrhoids

- rheumatoid arthritis and other inflammatory arthritides

- inflammatory joint disorders in general

- multiple sclerosis

- depression

Caution with Cryotherapy

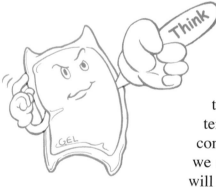

Several physical disorders necessitate caution when considering cryotherapy. In Chapter 6 we will be looking at conditions that involve contraindications to or require extensive adaptation of temperature therapy. In that chapter the conditions are discussed individually. As we are focused here on the use of cold, we will consider some general cautions for working with cryotherapy:

Once you have decided that cryotherapy is appropriate, there are some specific reactions to watch for and avoid. Frostnip (skin becomes pale, numb, and/or tingly) is the first stage of frostbite, which is damage to the skin and underlying soft tissues that results from exposure to severe cold. Any cryoagent with a surface temperature of less than 0°C (32°F) must be used with caution. Using some type of insulator (such as a towel) or lubricant between the cold source and the skin can help reduce the potential for damage.

Cold can be applied over a cast, but it must be done in a way that prevents the cast from becoming wet. For example, the cast can be covered in an airtight plastic bag before the application is done.

Superficial wounds must be treated with caution. While some symptoms of acute injuries can be effectively addressed with cold applications, care must be taken with any open wounds to maintain hygienic conditions and to avoid disrupting an early seal by wetting it.

Individuals who are very young, very old, or immunocompromised must be monitored closely – cryotherapy treatments may need to be modified (using shorter, less extensive treatments) to accommodate body system fragility.

Because of the short-term increase in blood pressure during a full body cold treatment (caused by global vasoconstriction), it is important to supervise anyone who has high blood pressure or cardiac disorders; in more severe cases full body cold will be contraindicated. As well, when treating a large area or multiple sites with cryotherapy, keep an eye on the person's blood pressure to make sure that it does not increase above acceptable parameters when the cryoagent is initially applied.

If the person receiving the treatment has a condition that involves nerve conduction problems, it is important to carefully monitor the effects of treatment on the tissues, since sensation may not be accurate and protective reflexes may not function normally. This applies to both peripheral and central nervous system injuries and disorders.

If the person has a thermoregulatory disorder it is important to monitor her or him carefully to avoid adverse reactions to cryotherapy.

Now that we have examined the primary features of cryotherapy, we will move on to study the effects that heat applications can have on the body.

There is evidence that the sweat lodges of the North American First Nations people date back to 400 B.C. Sweat lodges were used right across North America, and while each tribe's procedures differed, their intentions were similar.

These sweat lodges ultimately promoted physical, mental, and spiritual health. Sweat lodges also increased group cohesion because of the camaraderie in the lodges. Often sweat lodges were connected with gods and creation. The Sioux saw the interior of a sweat lodge as representing the womb of Mother Earth, its darkness as human ignorance, the hot stones as the coming of life, the hissing steam as the creative force of the universe being activated.

Chapter Three

Physiological Effects of Heat

Learning Objectives

After learning the contents of this chapter, the reader should be able to:

- indicate the difference between warm and hot temperatures
- indicate the rate of burning with temperature that is excessively hot
- define passive derivation
- explain hydrostatic pressure's effects on body fluid re-distribution
- demonstrate an understanding of the factors that determine treatment effects
- describe the pain → spasm → pain cycle
- identify the direct and reflex effects of thermotherapy

Muhammad, the Muslim prophet, recommended that people take sweat baths, which brought the Islamic hammam back into vogue, replacing cold showers. Originally women were not allowed to be in the hammam, but when they finally were allowed to participate, this privilege became a right. In fact, if a woman were denied the right to visit the hammam by her husband, she had grounds for divorce.

Chapter 3: Physiological Effects of Heat

How does heat affect the body? Heat applications result in many of the same responses that a natural temperature increase (i.e., fever) causes, but these reactions can be controlled when intentionally induced. The length of a heat treatment influences the body's response to the temperature therapy: short applications tend to be stimulating, while longer treatments are usually sedating. Since most people naturally prefer heat to cold and tend to overuse it, it is essential for practitioners to understand its effects and proper therapeutic usage.

Warm and Hot

In using heat applications, it is important to note the difference between a *warm* treatment and a *hot* one. Warm includes treatments that raise the target tissue's temperature to between 33°C and 38°C (92°-100°F); hot is over 38°C (100°F). Caution must be taken with prolonged hot applications because of the large increase in metabolism they can cause, which can lead to overheating. Warm treatments, however, can generally be very long with no adverse effects. The increased heat during a warm application is usually sufficiently countered by the cooling mechanism of perspiration.

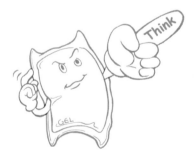

Caution must be taken with prolonged hot applications because of the large increase in metabolism they can cause, which can lead to overheating.

With hot treatments, the temperature difference between the application and the target tissue must be enough to increase blood flow and cell metabolism. In order to accomplish this increase, the tissues typically must be heated to between 40° and 45°C (104°-113°F). 40°C is greater than the average resting temperature of soft tissue and 45°C is less than lethal temperature. Between 45° and 50°C (113°-122°F), the rate at which burns occur doubles for every 1°C increase.

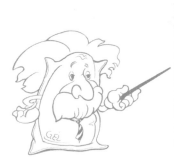

With hot treatments, the temperature difference between the application and the target tissue must be enough to increase blood flow and cell metabolism. In order to accomplish this increase, the tissues typically must be heated to between 40° and 45°C (104°F-113°F).

The heat treatments that we will be considering are superficial. Deep penetration of heat involves a specialized type of application, ultrasound, which moves through subcutaneous tissues to deeper structures. Superficial treatments tend not to penetrate more than about 1 cm (½") (Bélanger, 2002) because of the body's heat-losing mechanisms. The local effects of these treatments can sometimes be enhanced when used with other activities such as passive range of motion, stretching, and exercise. Heat and stretch together, for instance, decrease pain and spasms and increase range of motion more than heat alone or stretch alone. It is important to remember, however, that 'deep' and 'superficial' can be misleading because of the reflex effects of heat applications. Additionally, when large scale or multiple heat applications are used, the body can experience systemic effects, not just local ones.

Passive Derivation

The first effect that occurs following the application of a heat source is local vasodilation, the purpose of which is to allow heat to escape. Blood rushes to the body surface so extra warmth can be released and the tissue doesn't become damaged by excessive heat. This vasodilation response is a form of *derivation*, manifested as the movement of fluid away from the body core or from an inflamed or congested part toward the skin surface. When thermotherapy is applied, the ensuing warming of the tissue is perceived by the body in the same way as if it had become inflamed.

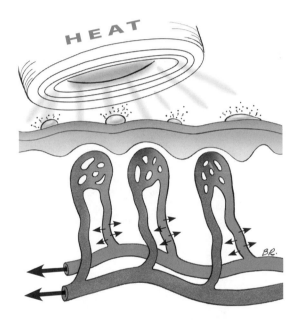

Figure 3.1:
Heat produces dilation of superficial capillaries, bringing more blood to the skin surface so excess warmth can be released.

In response to a heat application the derivation is *passive*, meaning that it doesn't require expenditure of energy. The blood that moves to the body surface does so passively as a result of *hydrostatic pressure*. Fluids exert an equal pressure in all directions on the walls of their container. When this type of outward pressure is exerted by body fluids in blood vessels and tissue spaces, these fluids will naturally tend to re-distribute outward from the region of higher pressure toward lower fluid volume tissues. So, if there is congestion in an area of body tissue, the fluid-filled region will experience more pressure than normal and fluid will tend to move outward from that tissue. When the blood vessels under a heat application dilate to cool the tissue, fluid from a higher hydrostatic pressure body area redistributes, helping de-congest the higher pressure tissue.

Figure 3.2:
Surface thermotherapy causes superficial vasodilation, which draws fluid out of a deeper area of congestion.

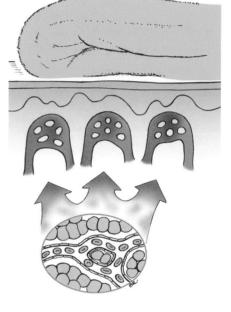

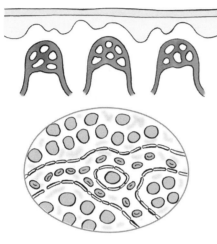

try this...
Next time you have swelling (somewhere other than your legs), or a headache, soak your feet in very warm water. See if your swelling decreases or if your headache lessens.

Factors That Influence Heat's Effects

The amount of heat that thermotherapy actually transfers to soft tissues depends on many factors. The greater the temperature difference between a heat source and the body, the more quickly and intensely effects occur – 'hot' is relative to body temperature. Also, the longer the duration of the hot application, the more the effects of heat will be experienced.

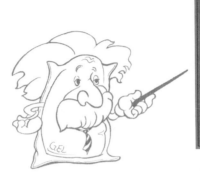

The greater the temperature difference between a heat source and the body, the more quickly and intensely effects occur – 'hot' is relative to body temperature.

The physiological changes that occur in response to heat depend on:

- the extent of the rise in tissue temperature

- the rate at which the heat is applied to the tissue

- and the size of the treatment area

Keeping in mind that an elevation in temperature increases local blood flow in order to remove excess heat, if the rate of temperature increase is very slow, the heat that is added could be counterbalanced by the incoming cooler blood. In such a case, therapeutic levels of warmth may not be obtained. Conversely, if the local temperature rises faster than any excess warmth can be dissipated, heat may build up and tissue damage may occur.

Qualities of the body part being treated impact an application's outcomes significantly. The larger the treatment area, the more widespread the effects. As well as the dimension of the body part being treated, its location greatly impacts the results. Subcutaneous adipose tissue conducts heat half as as well as skin and a third as well as muscle. This poorer conduction occurs because fatty tissue acts as a thermal insulator that reduces the transfer of heat to deeper tissues. It is important to keep in mind that the thickness of fat varies from tissue area to tissue area, so the same heating agent has different effects in different locations.

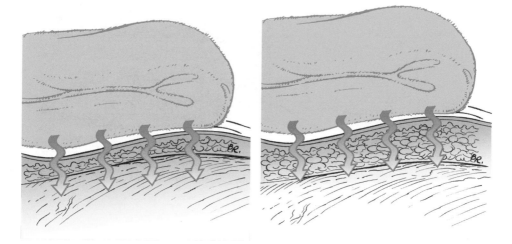

Figure 3.3: The amount of subcutaneous fatty tissue influences how much heat can penetrate into the tissues beneath.

Increasing the temperature to compensate for more adipose tissue may not always be a good idea because of the risk of burning the skin. However, heat transfer can be facilitated and accelerated by using a *coupling medium*, which is a medium or material paired with the temperature therapy to help tailor its effects to the goals of the treatment. For instance, as mentioned in Chapter 1, moist warm towels have a greater effect than dry towels of the same temperature because of water's conductivity.

Heating sections of the body can also effect changes in addition to those in the local tissues. The larger the volume of tissue treated by the thermotherapy application, the greater the likelihood that the effects will be systemic or reflexive as well as local.

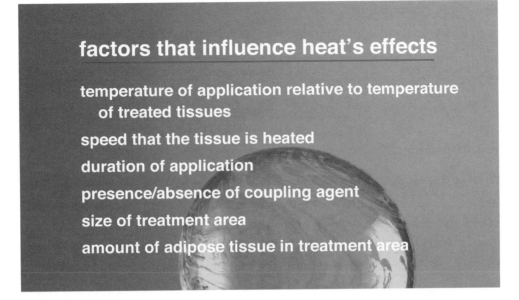

factors that influence heat's effects

temperature of application relative to temperature of treated tissues

speed that the tissue is heated

duration of application

presence/absence of coupling agent

size of treatment area

amount of adipose tissue in treatment area

Direct Effects of Heat

• increased metabolism of affected tissues

One of the key physiological effects of heat is increased metabolic activity. Stated simply, metabolism is the sum of chemical reactions in the body (the primary work of the cells); these activities occur more rapidly with elevated temperature. Van't Hoff's law states that chemical reactions increase two to

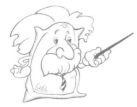

Van't Hoff's law states that chemical reactions increase two to three times for every 10°C (18°F) temperature increase. With sufficient, well tolerated heat, an increase in chemical activity increases oxygen and nutrient uptake in tissues, enhancing tissue health and performance.

three times for every 10°C (18°F) temperature increase. If tissue temperature rises past 45°-50°C (113°-122°F), burning will result because the mechanisms that prevent burning will not be able to keep up with thermally-induced damage. With sufficient, well tolerated heat, an increase in chemical activity increases oxygen and nutrient uptake in tissues, enhancing tissue health and performance.

- **altered cardiovascular dynamics**

Dilated vessels increase the rate of local blood flow, and increased metabolism increases the demand placed on the heart to deliver more nutrient-filled blood to the active tissues. With larger-sized thermotherapy applications, these effects in combination can be substantial enough to increase the return of blood to the heart, affecting *cardiac output* (the amount of blood pumped out by the heart per minute). The pulse rises about 6-10 beats per minute for every core temperature increase of 1°. This effect is strongest initially, since over time the individual usually relaxes under the influence of the thermotherapy and sympathetic nervous system activity decreases, resulting in a slower, deeper heart beat.

As well, large applications of heat create movement of blood from the core circulation into tissue beds. When there is a net shift of blood into the peripheral tissue beds, the pressure in the core circulation goes down, tending to normalize or reduce blood pressure. However, the initial effect, caused by an immediate increase in blood flow to the heart before there is time to achieve the counterbalancing peripheral hyperemia, can produce a quick rise in blood pressure.

Despite the potential for ultimately beneficial effects, these initial changes in cardiovascular dynamics caused by large-scale heat may not be well tolerated if the individual's heart is not completely healthy.

The pulse rises about 6-10 beats per minute for every core temperature increase of 1°. With thermotherapy, this effect is strongest initially, since over time heat usually induces relaxation and sympathetic nervous system activity decreases, resulting in a slower, deeper heart beat.

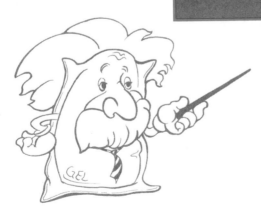

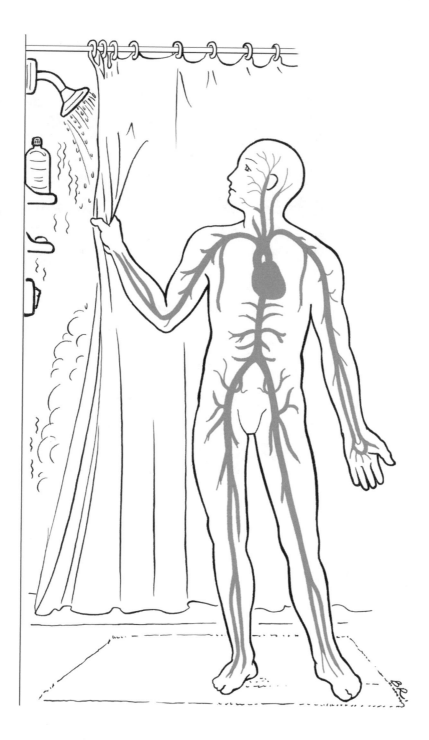

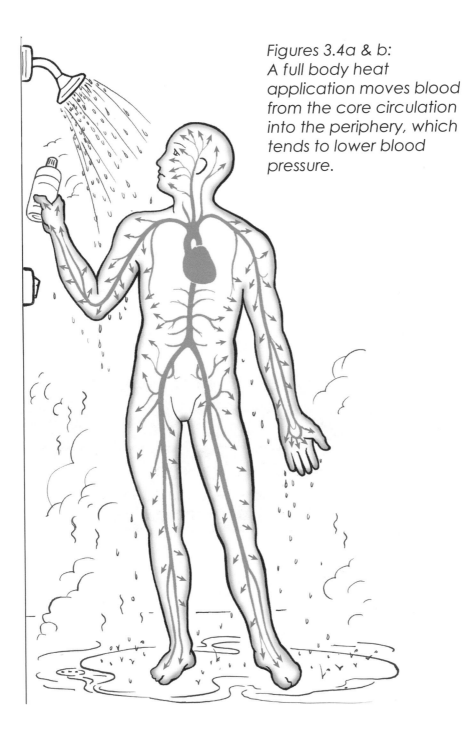

Figures 3.4a & b:
A full body heat application moves blood from the core circulation into the periphery, which tends to lower blood pressure.

- **altered blood dilution**

With the vasodilation and increased blood flow that follows application of heat, there is initial diluting of the blood (more interstitial fluid is mobilized) and increased blood volume. In counterbalance to this, *diaphoresis* (excess sweating) can cause fluid to leave the blood and make it quite concentrated (*viscous*). Fluid loss through perspiration necessitates replacement – usually by drinking water – so that good hemodilution is maintained throughout a long hot treatment and the person does not become dehydrated.

- **detoxification**

Perspiration increases the use of the skin as an elimination organ. This means that thermotherapy can have beneficial effects in reducing toxicity and supporting the other organs of elimination, especially the kidneys, lungs and liver. As well, metabolism in these organs tends to increase (a reflex effect discussed below) when their temperature rises, improving their performance.

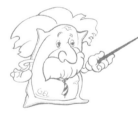

> Perspiration increases the use of the skin as an elimination organ. This means that thermotherapy can have beneficial effects in reducing toxicity and supporting the other organs of elimination, especially the kidneys, lungs and liver.

Heat also impacts on respiration rate. Breathing can be increased by a large scale heat application at a rate of 5 to 6 breaths for every 1° rise in temperature. This increased respiration helps blow off additional carbon dioxide.

As with heat's effects on the heart, however, these types of responses are more readily tolerated by organs that are healthy. Heat can also increase the volume of blood flow through the eliminatory organs, and it must be recognized that if there is impairment they may not always be able to handle the increase well. There will be more said in Chapter 6 about temperature therapy contraindications when these organs are diseased.

• direct effects on soft tissue structures

Other than reflex effects (to be outlined shortly), the impact of superficial heat on skeletal muscles is minimal. It is possible to effect more change to skeletal muscle tissue by coupling heat with exercise. Heat does directly affect joints, however, reducing their fluid viscosity and decreasing capsular stiffness. Thermotherapy applications that combine effects on muscles and joints can promote improvements in overall mobility.

Heat has a loosening effect on the strong connective tissue (*fascia*) that surrounds muscles and separates and supports other structures in the body. Fascia is not a very elastic tissue, so it has limited capacity for stretch. It can become stiff (*contractured*) and it can adhere to neighbouring structures. Heat can help loosen the fascia's ground substance, making its fibre network more pliable, and can also help 'unstick' it from other structures. Scars are fascial configurations as well. Heat is often used as part of treatment plans aiming to soften and stretch scars, improve their fibre alignment, and help reduce their tendency to adhere to tissues around them.

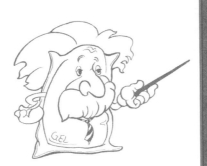

Heat is often used as part of treatment plans aiming to soften and stretch scars, improve their fibre alignment, and help reduce their tendency to adhere to tissues around them.

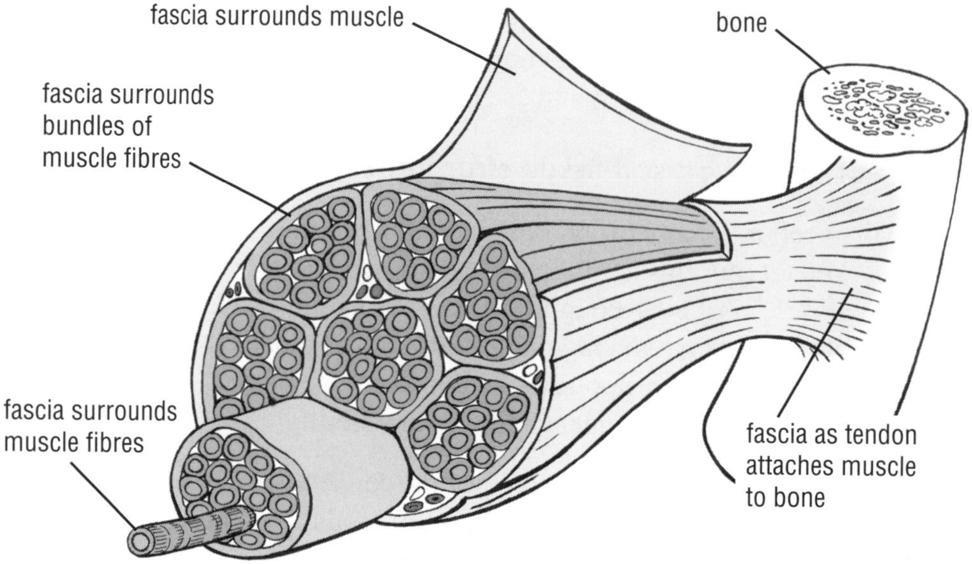
fascia surrounds muscle
bone
fascia surrounds
bundles of
muscle fibres
fascia surrounds
muscle fibres
fascia as tendon
attaches muscle
to bone

Figure 3.5: It is the fascial components of muscles, joints and tissue compartments that become stiff and restricted in contracture.

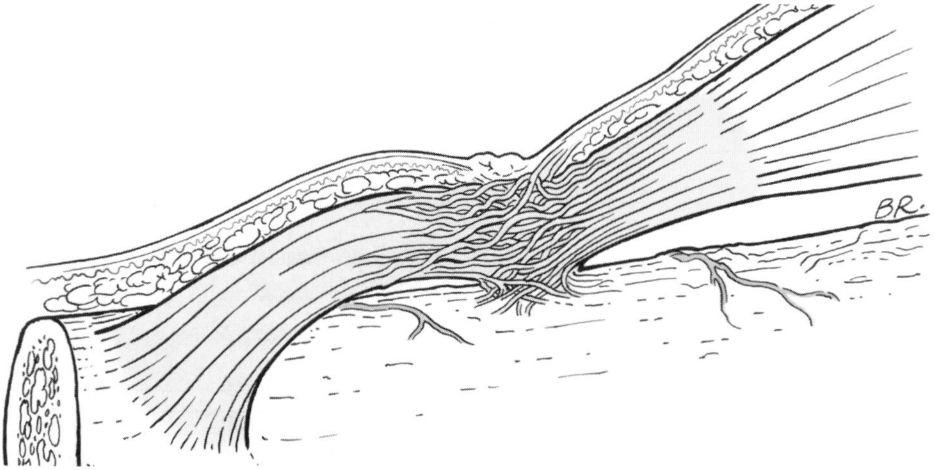
BR.

Figure 3.6: Scars are fascial structures that often have disorganized fibre direction, and that can adhere tissue layers that ordinarily move freely relative to each other.

direct effects of heat

area	effect
any	induces passive derivation; stimulates local metabolism and perspiration
cardiovascular system	increases demand on the heart but over time can produce a more relaxed heart by lowering sympathetic activation
	increases then decreases blood pressure
	increases then decreases blood viscosity
respiratory system	increases breathing rate and elimination of carbon dioxide
urinary system	aids due to increased excretion through the skin
joint	decreases stiffness
fascia	increases pliability

Reflex Effects of Heat

Brief heat applications do not tend to result in significant reflex effects. Longer treatments, however, can affect sites distant to or underlying the warmed surface area. There are a number of possible reflex effects on viscera. To give some examples:

- A long treatment to the abdomen reduces the blood flow to the intestines, decreasing motility and secretions, and therefore slowing digestive processes. Such a treatment can be effective in addressing intestinal cramping and diarrhea.

- Long hot treatments on the chest relieve respiratory congestion through derivation and relax the smooth muscle of the bronchioles, improving ease of breathing.

- An extended heat treatment on the pelvis relaxes the pelvic organs, for example, the uterus during menstruation onset. Blood vessels constricted by menstrual cramping dilate, so cramps diminish and menstrual flow is easier.

- The kidneys benefit from a prolonged heat application to the back or lower abdomen. The production of urine increases because of faster metabolism and more filtration in the kidneys. This thermotherapy can also help the ureters and the smooth muscle of the bladder wall to relax.

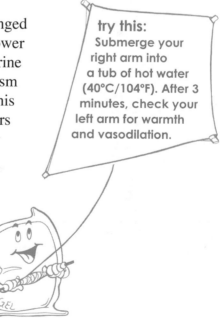

try this:
Submerge your right arm into a tub of hot water (40°C/104°F). After 3 minutes, check your left arm for warmth and vasodilation.

- A long heat treatment on the trunk also relaxes the bile ducts, which helps to relieve gallbladder conditions.

- Prolonged heat to one limb induces vasodilation in the contralateral limb.

The effects of heat on nervous tissue are not fully understood. We know that heat can have an *analgesic* (painkilling) effect. One theory is that heat applications block nerve impulses travelling to pain centres higher in the nervous system. Heat applications not only help diminish pain, they can also reduce muscle guarding. It is believed that heat elevates an individual's pain threshold, alters nerve conductivity, and decreases the firing rates of muscle spindles, which are the stretch receptors in muscles responsible for initiating protective reflex muscle contractions.

With a tissue injury (to muscle, joint, etc.) a cycle of pain→spasm→pain can start. Tissue vulnerability and the experience of pain result in muscle guarding that can persist well after the injury leaves the acute stage. Pain can raise the level of tone in muscles enough to cause spasm. Tension in muscles leads to compression of their intrinsic blood supply and drainage and to pressure on local nerves. These irritating events result in the muscles tightening and shortening further. Shortening of the muscles leads to restricted movement, which causes more pain, muscle spindle activation with smaller movements, and so on: pain→spasm→pain.

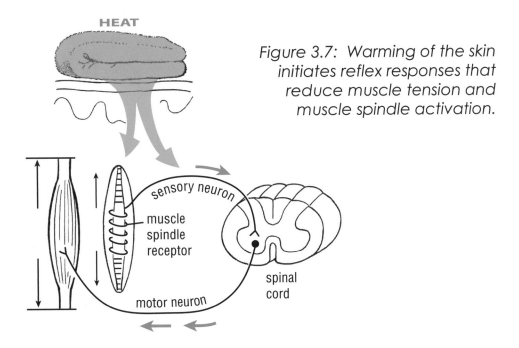

Figure 3.7: Warming of the skin initiates reflex responses that reduce muscle tension and muscle spindle activation.

79

Because superficial heat is likely unable to raise temperature inside muscles enough to decrease the pain→spasm→pain cycle, another mechanism must account for the reduction in pain. Heating the skin reflexively results in a reduction in certain types of *efferent* (motor) activity. Reduced efferent activity leads to less muscle spindle activation, which in turn decreases the *afferent* (sensory) nerve firing from the spindle. Ultimately there is a reduction of the motor firing that causes muscle contraction, decreasing the spasm.

This type of chronic elevated tone in muscles is characteristic of non-injury based cramps and spasms as well – these also tend to respond well to thermotherapy.

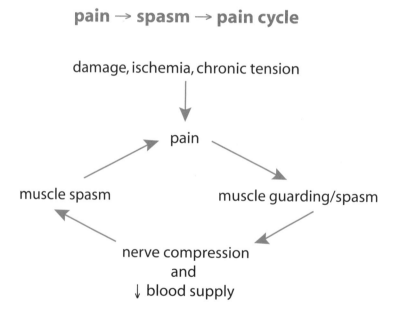

reflex effects of heat

prolonged treatment

area	effect
chest	relaxes bronchioles
pelvis	eases menstrual cramps
abdomen	decreases blood flow, motility and absorption in digestive organs
kidneys	increases filtration and urine production
trunk	relaxes bladder, ureters and bile ducts
extremity	vasodilation in opposite extremity
nervous system	analgesic, sedative
muscle	decreases pain→spasm→pain cycle
	reflexively increases flexibility

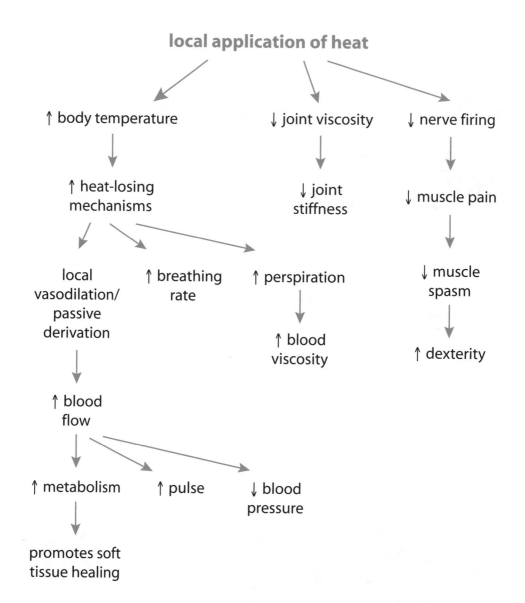

local application of heat

↑ body temperature

↑ heat-losing mechanisms

local vasodilation/ passive derivation

↑ breathing rate

↑ blood flow

↑ metabolism

↑ pulse

↓ blood pressure

promotes soft tissue healing

↓ joint viscosity

↓ joint stiffness

↑ perspiration

↑ blood viscosity

↓ nerve firing

↓ muscle pain

↓ muscle spasm

↑ dexterity

Indications for Heat Applications

There are many conditions for which heat is generally indicated. It is important to take a thorough case history and do an appropriate assessment in order to determine any cautions or contraindications associated with the person's case, but the following are conditions for which heat is typically helpful:

- promote injury/wound healing (after acute stage)

- non-inflammatory muscle pain, muscle spasm

- myofascial trigger point pain

- delayed onset muscle soreness (DOMS)

- conditions involving spasticity
  (note: most people with multiple sclerosis do not tolerate heat well)

- chronic tendonitis

- chronic bursitis

- scars

- soft tissue contracture

- non-inflammatory joint pain

- limited joint mobility, adhesive capsulitis

- poor mobility in general
  (to help increase stretch and range of motion)

- osteoarthritis

- rheumatoid arthritis and other inflammatory arthritides
  (not in flare-up)

- labour pain/perineal pain

- anxiety

Caution with Thermotherapy

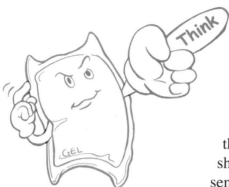

There are a number of physical conditions that require caution when considering using a hot application. Heat can be very soothing to people, but it is important during a thermotherapy treatment that the person not be allowed to sleep, as she or he will not be able to report sensations.

Any sensory or thermoregulatory disorders must be taken into consideration in determining an appropriate treatment, and careful observation of the tissue is important to avoid burns.

If a person is overheated before the treatment, or if a heat rub (e.g., A535) was recently used on the target area, time must be allowed for its effects to subside to avoid excessive local vasodilation.

If the individual is dehydrated (for example, at a sporting event), she or he must rehydrate prior to a thermotherapy application. The perspiration caused by a heat application will further dehydrate the person, so making sure fluids are replenished beforehand is important if using thermotherapy is indicated.

Heat increases demand on the cardiovascular, renal and respiratory systems, so it is necessary to evaluate the tolerance of the client. When disorders of these systems are present, heat applications often need to be modified to make them less intense.

Heat must be used with caution on a person who has a bleeding disorder such as hemophilia, or who has undergone prolonged steroid use. Either of these conditions can lead to an increase in the frailty of the capillaries, and heat can further tax those capillaries.

People with diabetes mellitus or peripheral vascular disease must be monitored carefully with thermotherapy because of compromised circulation in the extremities. Thermotherapy can put more strain on the peripheral blood vessels, so modification of the chosen application may be necessary. As well, individuals with these conditions tend to have accompanying sensory impairment and often cannot give accurate feedback about heat intensity.

Caution must be exercised when applying heat over the abdomen or pelvic area of a pregnant woman. A significant increase in the maternal body temperature may have negative effects on fetal growth and development.

Now that we have a good understanding of the effects of cryotherapy and thermotherapy on the body, let's look at what happens when they are combined in the same treatment.

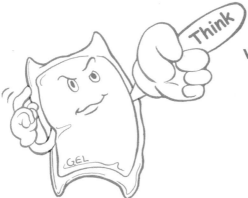

People with diabetes mellitus or peripheral vascular disease must be monitored carefully with thermotherapy because of compromised circulation in the extremities.

"We all know how man came into being. Man was created when God took a bania and sweated profusely."

Russian sorcerer, 1071

The Russian bath, or *bania*, was filled with hot steam. People anointed themselves with tallow and lashed themselves with young reeds to stimulate circulation. After being in the steam, they finished off in cold water or with a roll in the snow.

Chapter Four

Physiological Effects of Contrast

Learning Objectives

After learning the contents of this chapter, the reader should be able to:

- define contrast treatments

- demonstrate an understanding of vascular flush

- identify the minimum temperature differential that must be used for effective contrast temperature therapy

- identify suitable time ratios for different treatment needs

- describe how to end a contrast treatment appropriately

- explain indications and cautions for alternating treatments

Turkish baths are heated by hot dry, not moist, air. People go into three rooms of increasing heat, and often repeat the process with a cool swim or shower in between. The bath is followed by a massage and a full body wash, and concludes with a long period of relaxation in a cool room.

Chapter 4: Physiological Effects of Contrast

As we have discussed in the two previous chapters, heat and cold each have their own effects on the body. The range of therapeutic usage of these effects can be further expanded when heat and cold are used alternately on the same tissue, in what is referred to as alternating or contrast treatments.

Contrast applications enhance peripheral blood flow because they take advantage of the primary effects of both heat and cold, alternating local derivation and retrostasis (vasodilation and vasoconstriction). The result is known as a *vascular flush* or *circulatory whip* and can increase local blood flow by up to 100%. The derivation caused by the hot application brings fresh oxygenated blood that carries defensive and healing cells, and the cold limits local pain and reduces the build-up of edema and waste products. Because the temperature interchange creates opposing effects in circulatory flow, the effects of contrast treatments remain largely superficial and local, but they can work very efficiently to 'flush' the tissue. It is important to have a sufficient difference in temperature between the cryoagent and thermoagent to induce the desired effect.

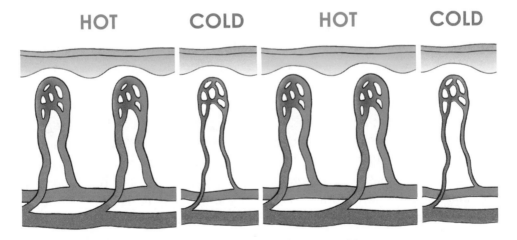

Figure 4.1: Contrast temperature therapy involves alternating use of heat and cold, producing cycles of vasodilation and vasoconstriction that 'flush' the tissues.

Contrast applications are much more effective at increasing circulation locally in a tissue area than heat or cold alone. Alternating treatments also reduce the possibility of having the increase in metabolism coupled with congestion that can occur with heat applications.

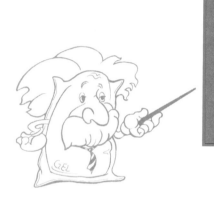

Contrast (alternating) applications are much more effective at increasing local circulation in a tissue area than heat or cold alone.

The duration of the components of contrast applications can vary, but an average guideline is a 3:1 ratio of heat:cold. For instance, a hot pack can be placed for three minutes, followed with a 60 second application of a cold pack to the same location. Generally this pair of applications is repeated six to eight times, making the entire treatment about 30 to 45 minutes long. When the treatment is combined with other modalities such as massage, it may be shortened to 3-4 applications. If a vascular flush with a reduction in swelling is the goal, always start with heat and end with cold. If the goal is ultimately to increase local circulation, finish with a hot application or a prolonged cold application, both of which cause derivation. Usually, however, contrast treatments end with brief cold to complete the 'flush.' If it is desirable to reduce the intensity of an alternating treatment, the temperature values can be reduced as long as a sufficient differential is maintained to ensure therapeutic effect. The minimum temperature differential must be 10°C (18°F).

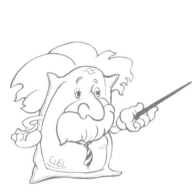

In a contrast treatment, there must be sufficient temperature differential between the thermoagent and the cryoagent to ensure therapeutic effect. The minimum temperature differential must be 10°C (18°F).

It is important to explain contrast applications to the individual receiving the treatment. People can be startled by a cold application on a warmed body part. Immersion of a body part into a cold bath after a warm bath can be especially disconcerting, so a thorough description of what to expect during the treatment helps minimize distress.

The 3:1 heat:cold ratio is a common guideline, but there are circumstances in which a different use of a contrast application can be helpful. If the individual has an injury or condition in the sub-acute stage of inflammation, where swelling is decreasing but still present, a higher proportion of cold to heat is appropriate. While heat is generally inappropriate on tissues that are inflamed, in this circumstance, when the symptoms are starting to abate, brief heat interspersed with longer cold (e.g., 5 minutes cold to 30 seconds heat) can increase the influx of fresh blood alongside of the flushing of wastes created by the alternation, helping speed the healing process. Likewise, when inflammation has subsided but swelling is still present, shorter heat with longer cold (e.g., 3 minutes cold to 1 minute heat) can be effective for facilitating the healing process while still reducing swelling and helping clear any remaining bruising.

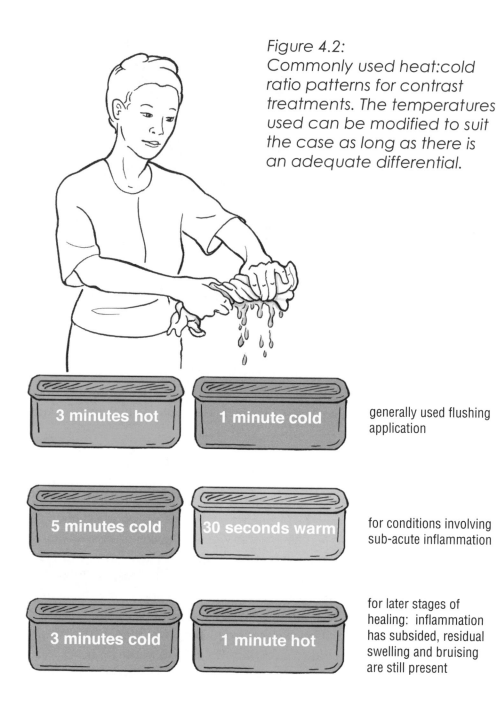

Figure 4.2:
Commonly used heat:cold ratio patterns for contrast treatments. The temperatures used can be modified to suit the case as long as there is an adequate differential.

3 minutes hot | 1 minute cold — generally used flushing application

5 minutes cold | 30 seconds warm — for conditions involving sub-acute inflammation

3 minutes cold | 1 minute hot — for later stages of healing: inflammation has subsided, residual swelling and bruising are still present

contrast applications

contrast (alternating) heat and cold temperature applications cause vascular flushing (circulatory whip) because of alternating derivation and retrostasis

generally the heat to cold ratio is 3:1; ideally repeat 6-8 times

must have a 10°C (18°F) difference between the thermoagent and cryoagent

usually end with cold

other time frames may be employed depending on the needs of the tissue

the vascular pumping effect can be increased when paired with active muscle contractions

It was once believed that the effects of passive contrast temperature applications were similar to the vascular pumping action that results from a muscle contraction squeezing and releasing blood vessels. Evidence now suggests that an active contrast treatment is more effective than a passive one (Shankar & Randall, 2002), so the alternating treatment is often best coupled with active muscle contractions to enhance the vascular pumping.

Indications for Contrast Treatments

Conditions with a need for 'flushing' of the tissues, such as edema, are the most common indications for contrast applications. However, many of the (non-acute) soft tissue conditions that are addressed with cold or heat can benefit from a contrast application, so it is an alternative that can be considered in many cases, especially if the individual prefers it.

While heat is never applied to acute inflammation, alternating treatments can be very effective in addressing sub-acute situations and chronic ones involving unresolved edema collection or circulatory congestion. Always determine the best heat:cold ratio for a contrast application based on careful observation of the needs of the tissue.

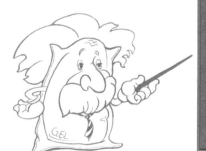

Conditions with a need for 'flushing' of the tissues, such as edema, are the most common indications for contrast applications. However, many of the (non-acute) soft tissue conditions that are addressed with cold or heat can benefit from a contrast application, so it is an alternative that can be considered in many cases, especially if the individual prefers it.

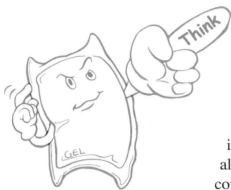

Caution with Contrast

Any of the conditions that require caution using either cold or heat must also be carefully monitored when applying contrast treatments. Peripheral vascular diseases are of particular concern because the increased circulation induced by alternating applications may overstress compromised vessels.

It is also especially important that there is healthy neural control of blood vessel wall diameters when contrast treatments are being used. Since the alternating thermotherapy and cryotherapy relies on normal vasoconstriction and vasodilation responses, nerve injuries or other causes of nerve impairment (for example, diabetes) can make contrast treatment inadvisable. If there is vasodilation without adequate vasoconstriction, the treatment may promote local congestion rather than relieving it.

Now that we have examined the physiological effects that cold, hot, and alternating applications have on the body, we will move next to look at how to determine the best treatment plans for individual clients.

Bene lave! (Have a good bath!) was a familiar greeting in the times of the ancient Roman *balnea* (baths). The giant baths, or *thermae*, of Rome were a significant part of Roman leisure time. There was an average of five bath houses per block and one *balneum* per 35 apartment buildings.

Roman baths were available in both salt water and fresh water. There were hot, warm, and cold baths, and the temperature of the rooms the baths were in reflected the temperature of the baths. The *caldarium* was the hot room, the *tepidarium* was the warm room, and the *frigidarium* was the cold room.

Chapter Five

Temperature Therapy Guidelines

Learning Objectives

After learning the contents of this chapter, the reader should be able to:

- take a case history and perform an assessment focused on temperature therapy issues and priorities

- explain and perform the skin discrimination test, the nail bed test, and patch testing

- define dosimetry and show how to make decisions about treatment components and variables

- explain how to determine a suitable treatment plan in cooperation with the recipient

- describe the rationale for and elements of informed consent

- identify important factors in preparing for and performing the treatment

- identify signs of discomfort or over-treatment and make adjustments

- explain how to end treatments appropriately

- discuss negative reactions, their causes, and appropriate responses to them

One of the oldest medical documents is the *Ayurveda*, which documents ancient Indian healing. It appeared in Sanskrit in 568 B.C. In the Ayurveda, sweat was considered vital to good health, and sweating was prescribed to give relief from colds, arthritis, headaches, and hangovers.

Chapter 5: Temperature Therapy Guidelines

Temperature therapy treatments can have powerful effects so it is essential to follow careful guidelines. Before the treatment is given, it is necessary to know what the presenting condition of the individual is, the treatment objectives, and which application will be most effective and why.

Case History

As with any type of therapy, it is important to take a thorough case history from the person receiving the treatment. All treatments must be adapted to the client, so be sure to take note of the individual's age, health status, and general constitution in addition to the specific concern to be treated. Check for the presence of conditions (discussed in the next chapter) that may contraindicate or require adaptation of temperature therapy applications. Discuss any such case findings, getting more details about the medical diagnosis, medications, restrictions that have been placed on temperature use at home, and so on.

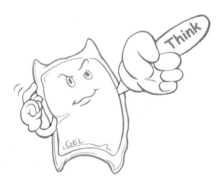

All treatments must be adapted to the client, so be sure to take note of the individual's age, health status, and general constitution in addition to the specific concern to be treated.

In conjunction with the recipient, determine the treatment priorities and which method(s) of addressing them best suits the particular needs of the client. A clear plan must be determined regarding how to check that the therapeutic goals are matched by the actual results, for example: Is range of motion improved? Is inflammation reduced? Has pain decreased?

Ensure that you understand the nature of the presenting symptom(s) and wherever possible, their cause(s). Ask about how the condition affects activities of daily living (ADL). If there is inflammation, it is important to know which stage of the inflammatory process the tissue is in. If there is pain, is the cause a primary or secondary concern? Is the pain local or referred or both? Ask questions to ensure you have the information you need that the client can provide, and so that you can proceed to conduct an appropriate assessment.

Assessment

Taking into account medical diagnoses and evaluations from other health care practitioners, it is still necessary to assess from your own professional perspective which area or areas of the body need to be addressed by the treatment and the status of the tissues relative to the treatment choices available. As with any therapy, it is crucial to gain as much understanding as you can of the presenting condition and the person's general health before deciding on a temperature therapy treatment.

Inspect and palpate the skin of the proposed treatment area(s), checking for tissue health, colour, swelling, sores, scars, and any other finding that might be relevant to your treatment decisions. The presence of any of these may alter the treatment plan. For example, edematous tissue does not typically receive heat or may require an adapted contrast protocol; open wounds/sores must be treated with caution to avoid wetting them, spreading infection or

> **Inspect and palpate the skin of the proposed treatment area(s), checking for tissue health, colour, swelling, sores, scars, and any other finding that might be relevant to your treatment decisions.**

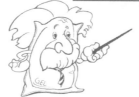

impairing healing; and scars may require their own specific treatment plan, which will vary depending on how recent they are.

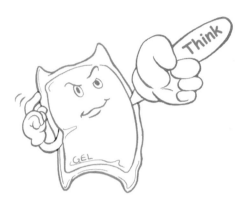

Keeping in mind the person's age, general health, and the presence of specific conditions, assess the tissues for specifics that arise from the case history. For example, if the individual has diabetes, you will want to look at both sensation and vascular sufficiency, especially if the target tissue is in the limbs. If the person is older, indications of reduced tissue health and poor circulation should be checked for.

- ## Skin Discrimination Test

If you have reason to believe the person receiving the treatment may have impaired sensation, especially for heat, perform a *skin discrimination test*. When someone has impaired sensory function, she or he is less able to accurately sense and report temperature, which increases the risk of burns or frostbite.

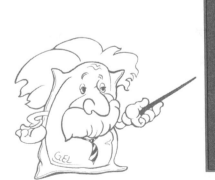

If you have reason to believe the person receiving the treatment may have impaired sensation, especially for heat, perform a skin discrimination test.

There are five degrees of skin sensory heat and cold discrimination: very cold, cold, room temperature, warm, and hot. They can be tested by using a set of test tubes filled with water at the different temperatures.

Very cold requires a test tube of water stored in a freezer, with a temperature of -5° to 0°C (23°-32°F). Cold is stored in the refrigerator and is 10°-13°C (50°-55°F). The room temperature test tube is stored in a container of water at room temperature and is 20°-22°C (68°-71°F). Warm is stored in a bucket of water with a thermal element to keep the test tube water at 33°-35°C (91°-95°F). Finally, a hot test tube is ideally stored on the wall of a paraffin wax unit and heated to 51°-54°C (124°-130°F).

Figure 5.1.

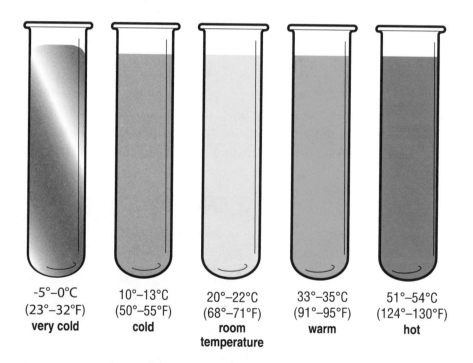

| -5°–0°C
(23°–32°F)
very cold | 10°–13°C
(50°–55°F)
cold | 20°–22°C
(68°–71°F)
**room
temperature** | 33°–35°C
(91°–95°F)
warm | 51°–54°C
(124°–130°F)
hot |

Explain the test to the person and describe the five temperature possibilities. Position the individual comfortably and uncover the skin area to be tested. Ask the person to close her or his eyes or look away so the test tube choices cannot be seen. Randomly apply the test tubes lightly to the potentially impaired area for 10 seconds each. Ask the person what temperature she or he perceives and determine if the response is accurate.

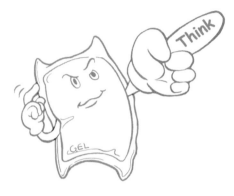

If the tissue sensation seems to be impaired, you may need to modify the treatment by shortening the duration or choosing a more moderate temperature. If you decide it is appropriate to proceed without modifying the treatment, you must be especially observant of the tissue's reactions to the temperature therapy application. Where the sensory experience of the client is not dependable, your close observation of indicators such as tissue colour is the key safety factor. When in doubt, you may want to perform a 'patch test' by applying the intended temperature application to a very small part of the tissue and observing how it responds.

skin discrimination test

intensity	temperature	storage
very cold	-5 to 0ºC (23-32 ºF)	freezer
cold	10-13ºC (50-55 ºF)	refrigerator
room temperature	20-22ºC (68-71 ºF)	room temperature water
warm	33-35ºC (91-95 ºF)	warm water
hot	51-54ºC (124-130 ºF)	hot wax

have person close eyes or turn head so as not to see the test
randomly apply test tubes for 10 seconds each
assess responses

• Nail Bed Test

Applying pressure to the bed of a fingernail or toenail compresses its blood vessels, decreasing local blood flow and making the compressed section turn white. Releasing the pressure allows blood flow to resume and the tissue to return to its normal colour. If uncertain about a client's tolerance for temperature therapy because she or he has a mild to moderate peripheral vascular disorder, or if you suspect vascular deficiency, you can get a sense of how the extremity circulation is working by doing the *nail bed test*.

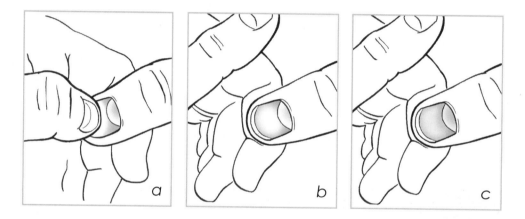

Figure 5.2: Performing the nail bed test involves compressing the tissue under the nail, and then releasing the pressure and observing how long it takes the tissue to return to normal.

Perform the nail bed test by itself and then during a 'sample' cold treatment to assess the person's normal recovery time. For example, you can place a hand or foot in a cold bath of 5°C (41°F) for 3 minutes as a test application. Remember to make sure that the person is not chilled to begin with.

When you apply pressure on the person's nail bed, be sure to support the palm of the hand or the sole of the foot well so you don't pinch the finger or toe. If the compressed tissue does not become pink within 2 seconds of being released during the cold application, the person may have an abnormal peripheral vascular response.

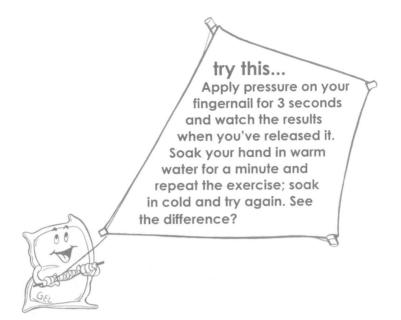

try this...
Apply pressure on your fingernail for 3 seconds and watch the results when you've released it. Soak your hand in warm water for a minute and repeat the exercise; soak in cold and try again. See the difference?

If cold treatments are indicated for the individual's presenting complaint, for example, with a diabetic with an acute ankle sprain, close observation of tissue reactions is essential. If there has not already been a diagnosis of peripheral vascular disease, medical investigation should be recommended and should take place before you proceed with cryotherapy. The nail bed test can also be used as a check during treatments when the client has compromised circulation.

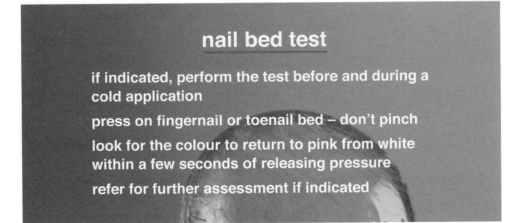

nail bed test

if indicated, perform the test before and during a cold application

press on fingernail or toenail bed – don't pinch

look for the colour to return to pink from white within a few seconds of releasing pressure

refer for further assessment if indicated

• Patch Testing

If, for any reason, you have doubts or concerns about how the individual's tissues may react to your proposed treatment, you can consider using a *patch test* to elicit responses in a small tissue area. Apply a small sample application of the temperature(s) or agent you are proposing to use and carefully observe the responses. Depending on the circumstance, you may also choose to wait until the next appointment to see how well the tissues returned to normal or if there were any overly prolonged effects.

> If, for any reason, you have doubts or concerns about how the individual's tissues may react to your proposed treatment, you can consider using a patch test to elicit responses in a small tissue area.

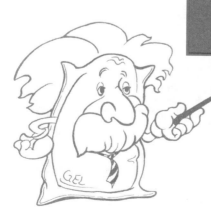

case history and assessment summary

take a case history and review it with the client

ask questions to elicit information so that you can understand the presenting complaint, including symptoms and their causes, status of the tissues, effect on ADL, etc.

identify and discuss any elements in the case that could involve contraindications or treatment plan adaptations

determine therapeutic goals and how to evaluate success in achieving them

perform a physical assessment to obtain the next stage of information and confirm/adapt treatment goals and plan

do a careful examination of the area of the body that you plan to treat

if there is known or suspected sensory impairment, perform the skin discrimination test

if there is known or suspected vascular insufficiency, perform the nail bed test

if further verification of tissue responses is desirable, do a patch test

Dosimetry

Dosimetry is the accurate determination of the appropriate 'dosage' of a treatment. There are a number of variables to be considered when determining a suitable temperature therapy application. Some of these factors can be controlled while some cannot.

It is valuable to consider both quantitative and qualitative information when deciding on a treatment. Quantitative data are measurable items such as the temperature to be used, the duration of the application, and so on, while qualitative considerations have to do with the recipient's experiential variables such as sensation. Some of the considerations over which you will have no control relate to the individual receiving the treatment, such as her or his age, health status, mental state, presenting condition, and general constitution. It is particularly important to take care when treating someone who is old, young, obese, ill, or sensorially impaired in some way. Regardless of whether the person has any impairment, however, all treatments should be adapted to the individual.

The remaining dosimetry factors to consider are more under the control of the practitioner:

1. Define the treatment area: The first decision is where you are going to treat. Also, are you treating the target tissue directly or via a reflex area? You need

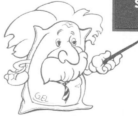

The larger the treatment area the more intense the effects and the greater the likelihood of systemic effects.

to decide on the size of the treatment. Generally speaking, the larger the treatment area the more intense the effects and the greater the likelihood of systemic effects. The overall resilience of the person must be considered alongside considerations about pursuing the agreed-upon treatment goals.

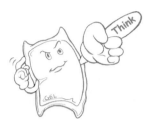

Keep in mind, too, that bony sites are more sensitive than fleshy ones, so the depth and volume of soft tissue and fat in the target tissue will influence your choice of application agent.

2.   *Application temperature (intensity)*: The next decision is what temperature(s) the treatment needs to be. Remember, what is significant in the intensity of a treatment is the temperature *difference* between the agent being used and the skin – the larger the difference the stronger the treatment effects. Once you have made a general temperature therapy selection (is heat, cold or contrast appropriate for this person and this condition?), you need to determine specifics: should the heat treatment be warm or hot, the cryotherapy cold or very cold, or what cycles and temperatures of contrast application are suitable?

> **What is significant in the intensity of a treatment is the temperature difference between the agent being used and the skin – the larger the difference the stronger the treatment effects.**

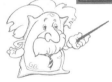

3.   *Therapeutic medium and use of coupling agents*: Complementing the temperature selection is the decision whether or not to use moisture (water) as a medium. A wet treatment penetrates deeper than a dry one, so this is a key consideration. It may also determine whether a coupling agent will be used with the application. If you choose to partner the heat or cold source with something, the type of material used is important. For instance, towels between a thermotherapy application and the skin will diminish the amount of heat exchange that will happen. Plastic laid between a paraffin application and a heat source like a hydrocollator pack, on the other hand, will keep heat in the tissue by reducing evaporation and heat dissipation, thereby creating a more intense and penetrating treatment.

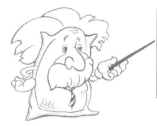

A wet treatment penetrates deeper than a dry one.

4.   Static or dynamic treatment: A decision must also be made about whether the treatment will be static or dynamic. A static application involves either laying the thermo- or cryoagent on the body part or simply placing the body part in the application (for example, an arm bath). A dynamic treatment involves movement of the medium, as in a whirlpool, or use of other techniques that enhance the effect of the application. Particularly with cold treatments, stimulating techniques can make the treatment more effective and more pleasant for people who don't like cold. For example, an ice massage is usually better tolerated than ice sitting immobile on the skin. Similarly, ice packs can be more easily tolerated when preceded or followed by percussive manoeuvres on the tissue being treated.

The speed with which the temperature agent produces its effects in the tissue is an important element of the treatment intensity.

5.   Speed of the temperature application: The speed of the treatment must be considered. Do you want to heat the treatment area gradually? Are you trying to cool the tissue rapidly? If you are using paraffin wax, are you going to paint the skin or dip the body part into the wax? The speed

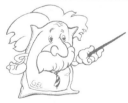

with which the temperature agent produces its effects in the tissue is an important element of the treatment intensity.

6.   *Treatment duration*: Whether the treatment is long or short makes a significant difference to the effects that will occur. Brief cold or heat applications tend to be stimulating (brief cold creates an influx of fresh blood and stimulates reflex effects; brief heat activates tissue metabolism), while longer cold treatments will depress tissue activities and longer heat will have sedative effects. As a rule, cold treatments should be no more than 20 minutes, with an interval of at least 30 minutes before another application. Heat applications should not exceed 20 to 30 minutes as there is no noteworthy increase in blood flow after 30 minutes and there is a risk of tissue congestion.

As a rule, cold treatments should be no more than 20 minutes, with an interval of at least 30 minutes before another application. Heat applications should not exceed 20 to 30 minutes as there is no noteworthy increase in blood flow after 30 minutes and there is a risk of tissue congestion.

7. *Treatment frequency and time of day*: The frequency and time of the application are important treatment planning considerations. The more easily fatigued or weaker the person is, the less frequent the applications should be. As well, the time of day has an impact, especially for individuals who are ill or debilitated. Treating at a time of day when the recipient feels strong makes for more effective outcomes.

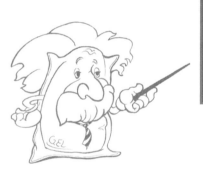

> **Time of day has an impact, especially for individuals who are ill or debilitated. Treating at a time of day when the person feels strong makes for more effective outcomes.**

8. *Use of additives*: Another variable is whether you are going to use additives to enhance the outcomes of your treatment. Do you want to use an essential oil in a foot bath? Is it appropriate to use sea salts with a cold treatment for this person? As with the temperature agent itself, you must understand the effects that any additives will have on the condition you are trying to address. (Additives are discussed in a later chapter.)

9. *Post-treatment activities*: Finally, you need to decide what activities are suitable after the treatment is complete. Some people rest after temperature therapy, some receive massage or other therapies, and some do

some form of exercise. The specific post-application activities are at the discretion of the therapist and the individual when they decide upon the treatment plan, but should follow these general guidelines:

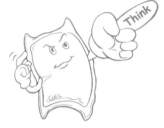

• After a short cold treatment the person should engage in active exercise suited to the circumstance or passive exercise such as massage, the purpose being to normalize blood flow into the chilled tissue.

• After a long treatment, whether hot or cold, the person should rest prior to exercise, receiving other treatments, or resuming routine activities. After cold treatments the therapist should ensure that the recipient does not become chilled while resting.

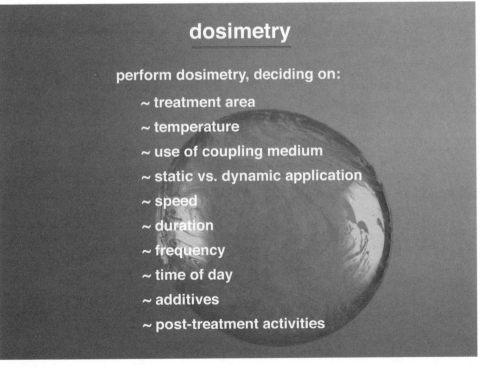

dosimetry

perform dosimetry, deciding on:

~ treatment area

~ temperature

~ use of coupling medium

~ static vs. dynamic application

~ speed

~ duration

~ frequency

~ time of day

~ additives

~ post-treatment activities

Informed Consent

As with any treatment, nothing should be started until the therapist has received informed consent from the client. *Informed* consent means that it must be very clear that the recipient understands the treatment and why it has been suggested, and then freely agrees to receive the treatment. Having given consent, however, it is still the person's right to end the treatment at any time or not to follow through with an agreed upon treatment plan. If an assessment protocol is part of the determination about the treatment plan, informed consent must be received before the assessment starts, too.

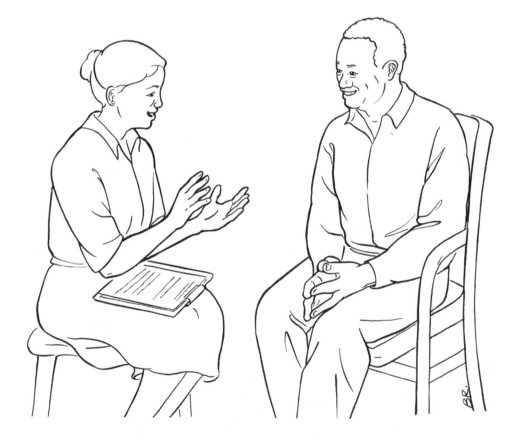

Figure 5.3.

The therapist must thoroughly explain the treatment that is being proposed, and why that particular treatment is considered most appropriate. The temperature, therapeutic agent, and equipment being used should be described and, if necessary, viewed or demonstrated. The time frame of the application should be discussed as well. Explain specifics about positioning and draping and modify if the person is not comfortable with them.

It is also important to go over the benefits of the proposed application, as well as any potential risks or adverse effects. Once you have covered all the aspects of the treatment, be sure to ask if the person has understood everything and if she or he has any questions. Once these questions have been answered, ask the individual for consent to proceed with treatment as described. Only then is it appropriate to begin the treatment.

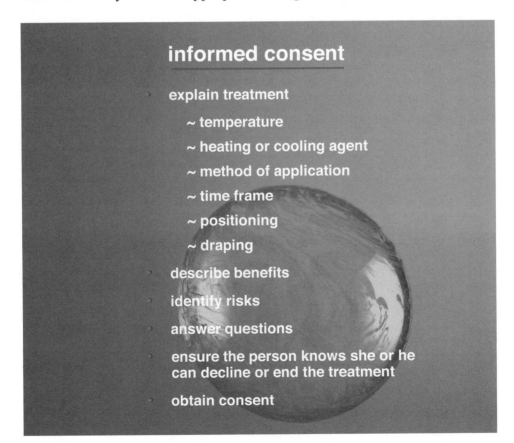

informed consent

› **explain treatment**

~ **temperature**

~ **heating or cooling agent**

~ **method of application**

~ **time frame**

~ **positioning**

~ **draping**

› **describe benefits**

› **identify risks**

› **answer questions**

› **ensure the person knows she or he can decline or end the treatment**

› **obtain consent**

General Treatment Guidelines

Once informed consent has been obtained, the treatment can start. It is usually best to have told the person ahead of time not to eat a large meal before a treatment, especially with larger scale or more intense modalities. There are several reasons for this:

- While digestion is occurring, substantial blood flow is directed to the digestive organs. Temperature applications that alter this may produce symptoms like nausea, and there is a risk of promoting abnormal local blood flow patterns.

- Digesting a large meal usually results in a decreased energy level – not ideal when the body is being asked to handle an intense therapeutic modality.

- After a large meal, certain positions appropriate for a temperature therapy treatment, such as lying face down, may be uncomfortable.

It is also best to have the person void her or his bladder before beginning the treatment so there is less chance of interruption.

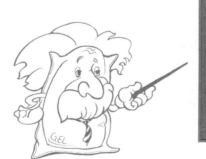

Tell the person ahead of time not to eat a large meal before a treatment, especially with larger scale or more intense modalities.

Always make sure that the treatment room is clean and calm. It should also be free of drafts because it is important that the person receiving the treatment not become chilled. If she or he arrives cold, use a warming application before starting the treatment. While this may seem obvious when planning to use cryotherapy, even with thermotherapy applications the person should not be cold before beginning the treatment since the temperature difference between the tissue and the heating agent will be greater than intended.

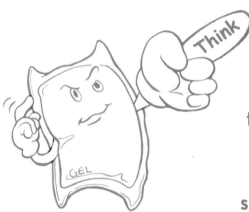

If the client arrives cold, use a warming application before starting the treatment. While this may seem obvious when planning to use cryotherapy, even with thermotherapy applications the person should not be cold before beginning the treatment since the temperature difference between the tissue and the heating agent will be greater than intended.

Be sure to maintain your equipment well, and check any materials you will need for an upcoming treatment to make sure that they are clean, working, full, and ready to be used. Before starting, ensure that everything you will need is readily available so there will be no need to leave the room. You should never leave an individual during a temperature therapy treatment. If you absolutely must leave, give the person an easy way to contact you (for example, a bell). This is particularly important if you are doing any type of full body treatment.

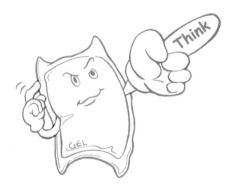

You should never leave an individual during a temperature therapy treatment.

Before beginning, ensure that the person or the target tissue is clean, as is appropriate to the size of the planned application. Have the individual remove any jewellery, particularly with hot treatments. If jewellery takes on the temperature of a thermotherapy or cryotherapy treatment, tissue damage can result.

Once everything is ready, position and drape appropriately. The person should be comfortable (anticipate the length of time to be spent in the selected position) and appropriately draped to preserve privacy while still uncovering the tissue(s) to be treated. The application can now begin.

During both local and full body treatments, watch the individual for signs of discomfort such as a very flushed or pale face, shallow breathing, or sounding weak or disoriented. Ask pertinent questions about the temperature, the person's overall comfort, any feelings of nausea or faintness, shortness of breath, any pain or unusual sensations, and so on. If the person reports – or you observe – any problems, make suitable adjustments. If you see any negative reactions (discussed shortly), stop the treatment. Many people believe in the adage 'no pain, no gain' and will not tell you if the application becomes uncomfortable or painful. This saying has no place in temperature therapy. Make sure your client understands the need to keep you informed.

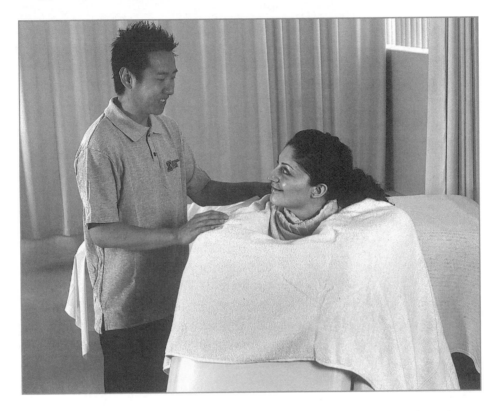

Figure 5.4: It is important to do regular comfort checks, especially when using intense large scale heat modalities, and to make sure that the client stays hydrated.

At all costs, avoid over-treating. With temperature therapy, more is definitely not better. A good rule to follow is *as cold as possible, as hot as necessary.* If you want the target tissue to be cooled, choose as cold a temperature as the individual can tolerate. The same is not true for heat, however. If the

119

person says that the temperature could be hotter, you still have an upper limit of heat that you can apply (45°C/113°F); anything hotter will cause tissue breakdown and burning.

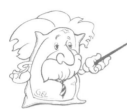

remember this:
As cold as possible, as hot as necessary.

• Local Treatments

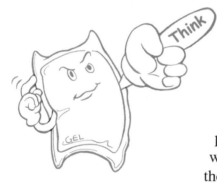

With local treatments, be sure to lay the heating or cooling agent *on* the person, *never under*. Placing a heat source under the body part traps in heat, impairs thermoregulation mechanisms, and greatly increases the risk of burning. As well, if the individual were to be positioned on the application agent, you would be unable to inspect the tissue during the treatment, which you should do periodically.

• Full Body Treatments

If you are doing a full body treatment, make sure to check the person's pulse and blood pressure regularly during the treatment. Remember, too, that with longer full body hot treatments metabolism increases but circulation slows. The increased body heat from faster metabolism is not easily dissipated – it is usually necessary to apply a cold compress to the person's forehead or neck to prevent overheating. It is also essential to provide water for sipping during the treatment to avoid dehydration. People receiving full body treatments should be monitored closely.

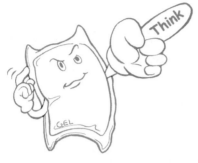

With longer full body hot treatments metabolism increases but circulation slows. The increased body heat from faster metabolism is not easily dissipated – apply a cold compress to the person's forehead or neck to prevent overheating. It is also essential to provide water for sipping during the treatment to avoid dehydration.

Ending a Treatment

Once the treatment is complete, examine the treated area for any adverse indicators. If there are any, inform the client and together decide upon an appropriate response, such as resting for a while or seeking a medical opinion. Make sure the person is dry and warm and follow up with the appropriate post-treatment activities.

Determine the efficacy of the treatment in meeting the goals you and the client have established, using the criteria you decided upon when you agreed to the treatment plan. Detail any goals that have been met, such as improvements in pain level, range of motion, swelling, and so forth, and any that have not. Document the treatment thoroughly, including the type of treatment, the treatment area, temperature(s), equipment used, duration, any additives, and post-treatment activities. If you are documenting a full body treatment, record the person's pulse and blood pressure before, during, and after the treatment. Note any responses from the individual, both during and after the application. Also, carefully document any changes in the skin, any unusual colour or swelling, for example, and any advice you may have given the individual if there has been an adverse reaction. Record your home care recommendations. You should also note any changes you and the recipient agree upon regarding the treatment design or goals.

general treatment guidelines summary

- pre-treatment
  - make sure the person hasn't eaten a big meal
  - have the individual void before the treatment starts
  - ensure equipment is well maintained and ready
  - have a clean, calm, prepared treatment space
  - ensure the room is warm enough and draft-free

- during the treatment
  - do not leave the person unattended
  - lay the heating or cooling agent <u>on</u> the person
  - ask relevant questions, check the tissue
  - during a full body treatment, check the pulse and blood pressure regularly
  - during a hot full body treatment, apply a cold compress to the head/neck and provide water to drink
  - use the nail bed test as a check if the person has a peripheral vascular disorder
  - stop the treatment if negative reactions occur

- post-treatment
  - when the treatment is finished, examine the tissue
  - follow up with appropriate post-treatment activities
  - determine what effects the treatment has had
  - document the treatment thoroughly, including both the individual's experience and your observations
  - record any home care recommendations
  - note any proposed changes to the treatment plan

Negative Reactions

A negative reaction is a response to the treatment that is unexpected and undesirable. Negative reactions are most likely to occur during:

- a hot or contrast treatment

- a treatment of any temperature that is too long, including excessive contrast applications

- a treatment of any temperature that is too short or incomplete

- a treatment where the person was chilled when the treatment began

- a type of treatment for which the person is too tired or too weak/debilitated

- a treatment that is too intense for someone not used to temperature therapy treatments

Common Signs and Symptoms of Negative Reactions

Symptoms of negative reactions in the skin and subcutaneous tissues most commonly involve:

- tissue discolouration or any unusual colour indicating poor local blood flow

- heightened sensitivity, paraesthesias (abnormal sensations), pain or itchiness

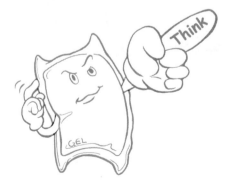

In the skin and subcutaneous tissues, negative reactions most commonly involve:

- tissue discolouration
- increased sensitivity, altered sensation or pain

Generalized signs and symptoms most commonly include:

- shivering

- dizziness

- low or high blood pressure

- headache

- nausea

- hyperventilation

- disorientation

- feeling faint

- other feelings of illness

Types of Negative Reactions

The four main types of negative reactions are:

• Arterial

In *arterial* negative reactions, the skin appears marble-like, with red and white blotches. The blotchy colour is due to the inability of the arteries to handle the increased blood flow caused by derivation. In a normal reaction to thermotherapy, the skin will redden to a consistent colour; in a normal reaction to cryotherapy, the skin will be red initially, and then turn pale after a prolonged application.

> In a normal reaction to thermotherapy, the skin will redden to a consistent colour; in a normal reaction to cryotherapy, the skin will be red initially, and then turn pale after a prolonged application.

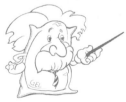

The arterial type of negative reaction is most common with contrast, intense heat, or long cold treatments.

• Venous

In *venous* negative reactions the skin appears red and blue, the red being the result of hyperemia and the blue caused by congestion. This response is due to the inability of the veins to cope with the increased blood drainage from the tissue. Venous negative reactions occur most often with long hot treatments.

• Paradox

A negative reaction is called *paradox* when the body responds in a way that is contrary to what *should* happen. For example, in response to a cryotherapy application the skin becomes pale, then red, then white as the local blood flow changes. In a paradox reaction, the skin may become pale then white and never become red, indicating that active derivation is not occurring.

• Combined

A *combined* negative reaction is a combination of two or more arterial, venous, or paradox reactions happening in response to a temperature therapy treatment. This type of reaction usually only occurs in people who have circulatory disorders.

How to Respond to a Negative Reaction

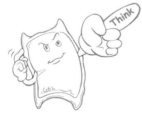 If a negative reaction occurs, *stop the treatment*. Give the individual sips of water, and have her or him rest comfortably and take relaxing breaths. If the person is pale, raise the feet to help the blood flow to the head; if she or he is flushed, raise the head to allow the blood to drain to the heart. Remember: *If she's red, raise her head; if he's pale, raise his tail.* If the person is chilled or shivering, cover with a blanket.

remember:
'If she's red,
raise her head;
if he's pale,
raise his tail.'

Specifically:

- For arterial reactions, stop the application and initiate a treatment to promote the gradual dilation of blood vessels, such as gentle massage.

- For venous reactions, stop the treatment and position the individual to promote drainage of the affected tissue. Once the person feels better and tissue colour begins to normalize, initiate gentle active exercise.

- For paradox reactions, stop the treatment and reassess the person's condition; possibly refer to a doctor.

- For combined reactions, stop the treatment and allow the individual to rest. Talk over the reaction in relation to the person's history with the condition. Medical consultation may be needed.

If the temperature therapy application was planned as a precursor to manual therapy, re-assess before starting any manual techniques. It may not be appropriate to proceed, or some techniques may be too stimulating for the individual at this time. You will need to wait a minimum of several hours before you can attempt another temperature therapy treatment.

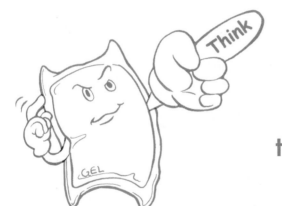

When a negative reaction occurs, you will need to wait a minimum of several hours before you can attempt another temperature therapy treatment.

negative reactions summary

- arterial

  most common with contrast, intense hot, or long cold treatments

  skin appears marble-like (red and white)

  person may experience cramping pain

  due to arteries not being able to handle the increased blood flow of derivation

  ⇒ stop the application and initiate a treatment to promote the gentle, gradual dilation of blood vessels

- venous

  most common with long hot treatments

  skin appears red and blue; the red is hyperemia and the blue is congestion

  due to the veins not being able to handle the increased venous drainage

  ⇒ stop the treatment and position the individual to promote drainage of the area; eventually initiate active exercise

- paradox

  the body responds in a way that is contrary to what should happen

  ⇒ stop the treatment and reassess the person's condition; possibly refer to a doctor

- combined reaction

  usually occurs in people with circulatory disorders

  ⇒ stop the treatment and determine an appropriate course of action

if there's a negative reaction...

stop the treatment

give the person sips of water

have the person rest comfortably

have the individual take several slow, deep breaths

evaluate the type of reaction

'if she's red, raise her head; if he's pale, raise his tail'

avoid further temperature therapy treatments for
several hours, and proceed with caution about
other planned modalities

consider medical referral

Our next subject area is contraindications to temperature therapy. This is closely related to topics covered in the present chapter, since the practitioner's goal is to provide effective and safe treatments. In some cases, people should not be given temperature therapy treatments, or the applications must be significantly modified. It is important for us to be able to identify such cases.

John Harvey Kellogg (1852-1943)
of the United States attempted to
show, in his graduate thesis, that
most diseases should be thought
of as helpful warnings rather than
enemies. He felt that symptoms of
diseases were the body's attempts
to correct a natural function that
had become disturbed, and
that pain was a prompting to the
sufferer to stop violating the natural
laws of good health. Kellogg
used water at his sanatorium in
Battle Creek, Michigan, to treat
infections and manage pain.

Chapter Six

Contraindications and Cautions

Learning Objectives

After learning the contents of this chapter, the reader should be able to:

- define the terms contraindication and caution

- identify the types of dysfunctions and disorders that raise concerns for temperature therapy treatment planning

- conduct effective discussions with clients to elicit information about elements in their cases that may constitute temperature therapy contraindications or require substantial treatment modification

- explain the ways in which several commonly encountered health conditions involve temperature therapy cautions or contraindications

- show an understanding of how to make appropriate treatment modifications

- explain some of the concerns regarding temperature therapy and medications

- list some effects of common medications that may skew or overlap with temperature therapy effects

"Anyone who believes that anything can be suited to everyone is a great fool, because medicine is practised not on humanity in general, but on every individual in particular."

Henri de Mondeville
(1260-1320)
French pioneer surgeon

Chapter 6: Contraindications and Cautions

In Chapters 2, 3 and 4 we looked at cautions for heat, cold and contrast treatments respectively. The purpose of this chapter is to discuss conditions, or categories of conditions, of which all therapists using temperature therapy need to be aware. In some situations substantial adaptation is necessary to modify the impacts of temperature therapy treatments on vulnerable tissues or body systems. In other cases, there are tissue states, diseases or disorders that make temperature therapy unsafe or inadvisable, or which preclude the use of certain temperatures or types of treatment. While heat and cold are very effective methods of treatment, neither is right for everybody.

What are Contraindications and Cautions?

There are conditions for which temperature therapy is inappropriate or potentially dangerous – these are known as *contraindications*. Certain physical conditions should not be treated with temperature therapy at all. Some contraindications are global to temperature therapy, while others are specific to heat, cold or contrast, or to specific types of applications.

The term *caution* is used to suggest that the practitioner must give careful consideration to how to design a treatment plan that is suited to the needs of a specific case. It indicates that the client's case history contains an injury or disorder, combination of conditions, or other elements that make applying temperature therapy more complex than usual. It means that significant temperature therapy adaptation is needed to ensure safety and an appropriate level of treatment intensity.

In addition to making good choices about temperature and type of application, the therapist is now considering how altered tissues or vulnerable organ systems will react to the treatment plan. This includes an understanding of how the person's condition(s) changes the way her or his body will react to temperature therapy applications. In part, this requires the practitioner to reflect on how the injury, condition, or disease has altered the affected tissues, and in part it requires a look at the person's overall health status and how the body is being affected by the stressors that are acting on it. Another element is the potential impact of a client's medications on physiological responses to temperature stimuli, a subject we will also discuss in this chapter.

There are conditions for which some or all temperature therapy is inappropriate or potentially dangerous – these are known as contraindications. The term caution is used to suggest that the practitioner must give careful consideration to how to design a treatment plan that is suited to the needs of a specific case. It means that significant temperature therapy adaptation is needed to ensure safety and an appropriate level of treatment intensity.

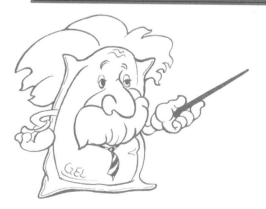

Temperature Therapy Critical Thinking

The first consideration is knowledge of the components of the case. A therapist should never do a temperature therapy treatment if she or he is unsure of the presenting condition(s). Temperature therapy can have very potent effects, especially if the body is not strong or resilient enough to handle them. So, the practitioner must do research to ensure sufficient understanding of what is occurring in the case. In some cases, this will include the need to get an opinion from the person's physician about temperature therapy judgment calls. If there is an uncertain situation with no diagnosis, the person should be encouraged to obtain the necessary medical evaluation before receiving temperature therapy.

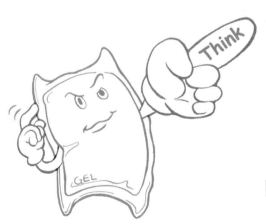

A therapist should never do a temperature therapy treatment if she or he is unsure of the presenting condition(s). Temperature therapy can have very potent effects, especially if the body is not strong or resilient enough to handle them.

Secondly, it is important to consider the status of the body systems that are the primary mediators of temperature stimuli. These include:

- *Cardiovascular System*: The heart and blood vessels are centrally involved in producing temperature therapy's effects. When cardiovascular structures are weakened or diseased, modification or avoidance of temperature therapy must be considered because of the changes in circulation that thermotherapy and cryotherapy induce, and the demands that these changes place on the heart and blood vessels. If an individual has cardiac or vascular insufficiency, there may be overtaxing of the diseased structures, or there may be an undesired increase or decrease in blood flow, edema or congestion, or stagnation created in the treated tissues.

- *Nervous System*: The central and peripheral nervous systems (CNS and PNS) are both key participants in the body's responses to temperature stimuli. The hypothalamus (see Chapter 1) is the central thermoregulator, and if it is malfunctioning temperature therapy considerations become much more complex. The autonomic nervous system controls functions such as heart rate, blood pressure, vascular diameters, breathing rate, kidney filtration, and so on, that are all involved in effective temperature therapy. The nervous system is also the mediator for a whole class of temperature therapy effects, reflex effects, and these cannot be employed effectively if the conduction circuitry involved is not functioning normally. Sensation is also a critical aspect of temperature therapy. While treatments can be done when there is sensory impairment, they require more cautious application and more careful monitoring because of the increased possibility of tissue damage. Some CNS conditions render the individual confused and unreliable, while others can change the person's perception of temperature and pain despite normal peripheral nerve function.

- *Respiratory System*: Breathing plays a role in responses to temperature, especially heat, since an increased breathing rate is one of the body's heat losing activities. Impaired gaseous exchange or breathing mechanics reduce the body's overall health, creating less resilient and less than optimally functioning tissue structures. They also tend to make the person intolerant of applications such as steams. As well, it is important to keep in mind the close interrelationship between cardiac and pulmonary functions. Chronic respiratory disorders tend to promote hypertension and congestive heart failure.

- *Kidneys and Liver*: The kidneys and liver each filter large volumes of blood every day. They are also key players in the body's system for eliminating toxins. If they are diseased or malfunctioning, they may be stressed beyond capacity by treatments that mobilize large amounts of blood flow. When these organs are diseased, there also tend to be a number of broader effects, including generalized reduced tissue health, and hypertension and overstress of the heart.

- *Skin*: Since the skin is the organ of direct contact for temperature therapy, skin injuries and diseases are another important group of conditions to be very aware of when choosing an appropriate treatment plan. Some applications may overstress early stage healing. Skin conditions may be aggravated by hot, cold, wet, or any sudden temperature change. Hydrotherapy may help spread infectious skin conditions. As well, the excess perspiration caused by a thermotherapy application can irritate many skin pathologies.

Next, the case information must be put together in the broader picture of the person's age and overall health status. A young, active, generally healthy person with diabetes, for example, is a very different client than an elderly, fragile diabetic with an amputation and severe cardiac and renal disease. The very young and very old should always be treated more cautiously, irrespective of specific health conditions. General fitness level and routine tolerance of temperature exposures are also important pieces of the case picture.

Medications

An additional consideration when working with people with health conditions is the medications they may be taking. Some medications will contraindicate some or all temperature therapies, and others will introduce a new set of cautions. They can substantially alter reactions to, or perceptions of, temperature stimuli.

Medications can also introduce new symptoms. They may create effects that can blur the known facts of a case. For example, is a specific new symptom a development in the person's presenting condition(s), a reaction to a temperature therapy application, or a medication side effect? Or is it perhaps a medication-induced abnormal or excessive reaction to the temperature therapy? As well, medications can make it more difficult to perform an accurate tissue assessment since they can suppress tissue processes, like the inflammatory response, or symptoms such as pain. It is also important to note that the long term use of many medications may adversely affect the kidneys and liver, which are the primary organs of filtration, and/or cause additional health conditions to develop in the body.

> Some medications will contraindicate some or all temperature therapies, and others will introduce a new set of cautions. They can substantially alter reactions to, or perceptions of, temperature stimuli.

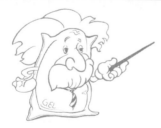

Sometimes medications cause effects that are not problematic, but that can skew the results of a temperature therapy treatment. For instance, ibuprofen, a commonly used anti-inflammatory, can cause an increase in perspiration, regardless of a thermotherapy application.

If the effects of a medication mimic common complaints such as headache, swelling, or muscle soreness, a temperature application may not be as effective as it otherwise would be in addressing such complaints. Be mindful, too, that more than one medication may be prescribed for a condition. For instance, muscle spasms may be treated with an anti-inflammatory and a muscle relaxant, both of which have their own unique effects.

Since some of the effects of medications could appear to be reactions to your temperature treatment, or could make planning an appropriate treatment or evaluating its efficacy more difficult, it is important to familiarize yourself with the mechanisms of action and common side effects of medications the client is taking. This information can be researched in texts or on-line; pharmacists are also very helpful and knowledgeable resources. When in doubt, the person's physician should be consulted.

When taking the health history, find out not only what medications the person is using and for what condition(s), but also when she or he takes the dosage. People can experience changes in mood, energy level, responsiveness, and communicativeness, all of which must be taken into consideration with a temperature therapy treatment.

The chart which follows is a list of common medication side effects. Recognizing that symptoms such as these may be medication-induced is an important first step in the process of differentiating medication-related changes from effects of temperature therapy applications.

> For a detailed description of classes of medications, their effects and uses, common side effects, and ways in which they can impact temperature therapy applications, consult *Massage Therapy & Medications* by Randal S. Persad, Dip. Pharm., RMT, published in 2001 by Curties-Overzet Publications, Toronto, Ontario.

common medication side effects

anxiety
bradycardia (slow heart rate)
back pain
blurred vision
breathing difficulty
bronchospasm
bruising
chest pain
chills
cold extremities
confusion
constipation
convulsions
cough
decreased sweating
depression
diarrhea
dreams - vivid
drowsiness
dry mouth
dizziness
dry airway passages
dysrhythmia
  (abnormal heart rhythm)
edema
facial flushing
fatigue
fever
hallucinations
headaches
heat stroke
hypertension
  (high blood pressure)
hypotension
  (low blood pressure)
insomnia
joint pain

light headedness
migraine
mood changes
muscle cramps
muscle weakness
nausea
nasal stuffiness
neck pain
nervousness
neuritis (nerve inflammation)
numbness
palpitations (irregular heart beat)
paraesthesia
  (abnormal sensation)
prolonged bleeding time
rash
restlessness
sedation
seizures
shortness of breath
slurred speech
sore throat
sweating
thirst
tiredness
tachycardia (fast heart rate)
thrombocytopenia
  (low platelet count, often
  leading to hemorrhage)
tinnitus
  (persistent noise in the ear)
tremor
urinary frequency changes
vomiting
weak pulse
weakness
wheezing

Contraindications and Cautions List

In this section you will find a list of conditions requiring serious consideration in temperature therapy treatment planning. Some are contraindications to thermotherapy and/or cryotherapy, while others require substantial modification of temperature therapy applications. Please be aware that although it is comprehensive, this is by no means an exhaustive list.

> *Note: When a condition appears in bold-face in the text, it is defined at another point in the list.*

- ## Allergies

Allergies are always a concern for practitioners and should be a routine part of case history inquiry. In the temperature therapy context, allergies are most frequently an issue with respect to additives (see Chapter 9). Some individuals also have strong reactions to some types of cleaning supplies, which might be relevant if the specific cleanser is being used on equipment such as steam cabinets or whirlpools.

- ## Angina Pectoris

Angina pectoris is most commonly caused by **atherosclerosis**, which can produce partial blockage of coronary arteries. Other possible causes are vasospasm or the presence of restrictive scar tissue in the artery wall. If the lumen (inner passageway) of an artery is adequate to allow sufficient blood flow for the needs of its part of the heart wall, there will be no symptoms. Sometimes what occurs is that the lumen is sufficient for some levels of activity but not others. When the heart needs more blood during physical exercise, emotional stress, and so on, inadequate perfusion creates cardiac pain. This pain is experienced sub-sternally, across the chest, and often down one or both arms or up into the jaw. The pain subsides when the demand level goes back to normal. One potential trigger of an angina attack that is especially relevant to temperature therapy is sudden changes in the temperature of the individual's body/environment, since this causes large-scale shifts in blood flow and blood pressure to which the heart must adapt.

- ## Arterial Insufficiency

Arterial insufficiency is inadequate blood flow in the arteries that can be caused by a variety of problems, several of which (for example, **atherosclerosis**, **diabetes**, **Buerger's Disease**), are discussed further on in this list. The primary effect of arterial insufficiency is *ischemia* (inadequate blood supply) and a resulting decline in tissue health. When the insufficiency is the result of an arterial pathology, as opposed to an issue like muscle tension impairing local blood flow, a thermotherapy application could place too much demand on the affected artery(ies) and exacerbate the condition.

- ## Arteritis/Phlebitis

Arteritis is an inflammatory condition of the arteries, which can occur independently or in conjunction with another pathology. *Phlebitis* is the inflammation of a vein, which is often accompanied by a **thrombus** (similar to a clot), in which case the condition is called **thrombophlebitis**. Temperature therapy, especially on-site heat, can aggravate these conditions because of the inflammation. Temperature therapy effects that promote increased blood flow through the affected vessels may also aggravate their condition or lead to increased pain and tissue congestion, so modification is required if thermotherapy or cryotherapy is indicated.

- ## Arteriosclerosis

Arteriosclerosis is the thickening, loss of elasticity, and calcification of arterial walls resulting in reduced tissue perfusion (supply of fresh arterial blood to match the tissue's current need). Arteriosclerosis is a common cause of **arterial insufficiency**, especially in the elderly. Care must be taken with temperature therapy, particularly large scale heat or contrast applications, because they require changes in blood vessel diameter that may not be possible. A generalized reduction in arterial elasticity promotes hypertension and stresses the heart, so modifications related to these systemic factors are likely to be relevant to the case. Severe arteriosclerosis is a contraindication for all but very mild local temperature therapy applications.

- **Asthma**

Asthma is a respiratory condition characterized by episodes of bronchiolar constriction, copious mucus production, and formation of mucus plugs in the small respiratory passages. Sometimes the trigger is exposure to an allergen or irritating substance, and in other cases it is not clear why the attacks occur. During an attack the individual experiences severe, potentially dangerous shortness of breath (**dyspnea**). Unless expressly recommended by a physician, temperature therapy is contraindicated during an attack.

Sometimes people with asthma are also chronically short of breath, and in general they tend to want to avoid situations that may challenge their breathing capacity. In the temperature therapy context, these situations would most commonly include larger hot applications, steams, applications that involve significant pressure or weight on the chest (such as a whirlpool or a large hydrocollator pack), or extreme temperature changes. Different individuals will have different tolerance levels. Asthma is also stressful on the heart, so cardiovascular concerns may be a factor in some cases. Medications can also be an important consideration.

- **Atherosclerosis**

Atherosclerosis is the most common type of **arteriosclerosis** and is a leading cause of death from heart attack, stroke, and other complications. Plaques of cholesterol and fats form in the inner layers of the arteries, leading to calcification and a loss of elasticity. These plaques can be unstable, releasing embolic debris, and are frequent sites of **thrombus** formation. A thrombus can occlude (block) the artery, killing the tissue it supplies, or can break away from the blood vessel wall and occlude a blood vessel in another location such as a lung or the brain. Since atherosclerosis ends to be systemic, and is so common in the client population, it is important to determine the degree of risk associated with a specific case. Many individuals with mild atherosclerosis (often undiagnosed) routinely take hot baths or showers, or swim in cool swimming pools. On the other hand, people with severe atherosclerosis have frequently been given a number of medical restrictions regarding hot and cold exposures. It is important to assess each case, taking into consideration condition severity, general health status, presence of hypertension and/or heart failure, activities of daily living, and any restrictions and/or medications prescribed by a doctor. Keep in mind that a history of heart attack, **angina pectoris**, or stroke is almost always an atherosclerosis diagnosis, and that diabetics are prone to more severe atherosclerosis development.

- **Athlete's Foot**

Athlete's foot is *tinea pedis*, which is a fungal infection of the skin of the foot. Heat tends to aggravate this condition.

- **Bleeding/Hemorrhage**

A hemorrhage is internal or external bleeding, and is a term usually reserved for significant blood loss in a short period of time. Any tissue that is currently bleeding, has recently hemorrhaged, or has a strong potential to bleed is not a good candidate for temperature therapy, especially hot or contrast treatments. Cold may be suitable in some cases, for example with recent contusions, but when there is active bleeding the practitioner must assume a general contraindication and take pains to verify that any temperature therapy is in fact appropriate. The risk is of promoting more hemorrhage or of impairing mechanisms that stop bleeding.

With bruises, which are the result of blood seepage into tissue after an injury, temperature therapy should be appropriately geared to the stage of resolution of the bruise.

- **Bronchitis, Chronic**

Chronic bronchitis, which is usually caused by smoking or other long-term inhalation of damaging materials, involves loss of the respiratory tract *cilia* that clear passageways. There may also be an increase in mucus production by the glands in the trachea and bronchi, all of which results in chronic cough. People with chronic bronchitis often experience **dyspnea** and wheezing. While thermotherapy is often very helpful in reducing respiratory muscle tension and mobilizing secretions, there may be an intolerance of intense heat or steam environments due to the dyspnea. There may also be some degree of **congestive heart failure**.

- ### Buerger's Disease

Buerger's Disease is also known as *thromboangiitis obliterans* (*TAO*). This condition involves the inflammation of small and medium sized arteries and veins (**arteritis/phlebitis**), usually in the leg/foot. The intense inflammatory episodes lead to progressive destruction of blood vessel lumina, infarctions (tissue death due to loss of blood supply) and **gangrene**. There is also a high **thrombosis** risk. All local temperature therapy is contraindicated with Buerger's Disease unless specifically approved by the person's vascular specialist. With respect to treatment of other parts of the body, temperature therapy may be appropriate; cardiovascular status and medications must be taken into consideration.

- ### Burns, Blisters

A blister is a fluid-filled bubble in the skin. A burn is a heat injury which results in redness and possible blistering of the skin and damage to underlying tissues. Thermotherapy is a local contraindication to both blisters and burns, as heat exacerbates them both, as well as any inflammation that may be present.

- ### Cachexia

Cachexia is a condition of general malnutrition, including weakness and emaciation, which is generally secondary to severe or end-stage diseases such as terminal cancer or AIDS. Temperature therapy, if indicated, must be greatly modified to avoid fatigue or further stress of the organ systems. It is also important to remember that the individual has virtually no body fat to act as a temperature insulator. Mild washings or compresses may be soothing or appropriately energizing – most other types of applications may be too intense.

- ## Cardiovascular Disease

Many of the conditions discussed in this list involve cardiovascular disease or dysfunction. Since the cardiovascular system and its individual structures (heart, blood vessels) are primary mediators of temperature therapy stimuli, and therefore have extra demands placed on them, it makes sense that weakness or vulnerability of these structures will raise concerns about the use of temperature therapy. In some cases there is an absolute contraindication and in others caution must be exercised to achieve a safe degree of adaptation. This is particularly true with respect to the larger, more intense types of applications discussed in Chapter 8. In general, the concerns relate to:

- acute or recent conditions, for example *heart attack*, *stroke*, cardiac or vascular surgeries, where the tissue, blood vessels and/or blood flow may not yet be stabilized and the risk of **bleeding/hemorrhage** and **thrombosis** may be high

- conditions (for example, **congestive heart failure**, **angina pectoris**, **hypertension**) where overly intense temperature therapy stimuli might exceed the capacity of the compromised heart muscle to safely handle the additional workload

- high blood pressure (**hypertension**), especially if severe or unstable

- any inflammatory conditions of the heart or blood vessels

- any condition with a significant **thrombosis** risk

- ## Chemotherapy

Chemotherapy is systemic cancer treatment involving the use of a range of potent chemicals that usually have broadly generalized effects. In addition to knowing information about the cancer patient's case (e.g., stage, medical treatment history, which body tissues are affected, other medications being taken, current general health status), it is important to keep in mind that chemotherapies have a number of specific effects relevant to temperature therapy decision-making. These include: extreme fatigue/debility, toxicity, low blood cell counts, pain and nerve irritation, altered clotting, some degree of skin and small blood vessel fragility, and the potential for altered sensation.

There is also considerable stress on the vital organ systems, especially the heart, liver, and kidneys. Different chemotherapy agents have different effects, and individuals experience differing degrees of symptom severity. While chemotherapy does not contraindicate temperature therapy in an absolute sense, adaptations suited to the circumstances of the case must always be implemented.

- **Cold Hypersensitivity**

Cold hypersensitivity is an unusual, extreme sensitivity to cold temperatures, which can result in **cold urticaria**, *erythema* (redness, blotchiness), and pain or itching.

- **Cold Hemoglobinuria**

Hemoglobin is the blood protein that carries oxygen. Hemoglobinuria is the abnormal presence of hemoglobin in the urine and is associated with the development of severe *anemia* (insufficient oxygen delivery to the body's tissues). In cold hemoglobinuria, red blood cells are broken down in cold temperatures, resulting in a pathological release of hemoglobin. Cryotherapy is therefore contraindicated when an individual has this condition.

- **Cold Urticaria**

Cold urticaria is sensitivity to cold that is characterized by the formation of *wheals* (angry red skin lesions). Cryotherapy is contraindicated.

- **Confused/Unreliable Feedback/Unable to Communicate**

People who are confused or unable to communicate clearly cannot be relied upon to properly report skin sensations, so the risk of tissue damage with temperature therapy is increased. Temperature therapy is not inevitably precluded, but the practitioner must assume additional responsibility for closely observing tissue reactions and monitoring for signs of distress or negative reactions. It is usually best to introduce temperature therapy in smaller, milder formats and increase the intensity if it seems appropriate.

- ## Congestive Heart Failure (CHF)

Congestive heart failure is weakness of the heart in its role as a muscular pump. This is a chronic condition that may progress over many years; sometimes there are acute episodes if the heart becomes very overstressed. Chronic heart failure can be caused by any number of conditions inside and outside the heart, for example: heart attack, valve disorders, **hypertension**, **diabetes**, anemia, **atherosclerosis**, respiratory conditions such as **emphysema**, **kidney disease**, some types of **epilepsy**, full body **spasticity**, **chemotherapy**, and so on – the list would include any factor that damages or chronically overworks the heart. The practitioner must always consider the possibility or degree of CHF when the client's case includes a history of heart disease or potential extrinsic heart stressors.

CHF leads to inadequate oxygen delivery to tissues and reduced tissue health, systemic and pulmonary **hypertension**, lung congestion, and generalized edema. CHF can be mild, moderate or severe. Mild cases may be fine for many temperature therapy treatments; a moderate case could require substantial treatment adaptation; and a severe or unstable case usually contraindicates most temperature therapy applications, especially large scale or intense ones. It is helpful to consider the person's everyday temperature-related activities and tolerance level as well as any related medical restrictions. It is also important to keep in mind that the skin and other tissues may be significantly *dystrophic* (unhealthy).

- ## Cryoglobulinemia

Cryoglobulinemia involves the presence of cryoglobulins in the blood. A cryoglobulin is an abnormal plasma protein that typically dissolves at normal body temperatures, but separates and aggregates with exposure to low temperatures. These cryoglobulins can impair circulation in small blood vessels. Cryotherapy is contraindicated.

- ## Diabetes Mellitus

Diabetes mellitus is an endocrine disorder involving inadequate insulin production, release, or utilization; physiological processes are extensively affected by the resulting impairment of glucose use in the body, since glucose is a primary cellular fuel. Diabetes, especially Type 1 (*insulin dependent*) diabetes, raises a number of considerations for the temperature therapist. Firstly, it is important to be concerned about diabetic stability. In the insulin dependent diabetic, the person's insulin intake must be matched to the body's anticipated need. Activities that require substantial metabolic activity may increase that need beyond expected parameters. It is always a good idea to schedule temperature therapy treatments closer to the beginning of a new insulin injection period. The client should also be questioned thoroughly about regular temperature practices and tolerances and any history of destabilization with past temperature therapy or similar situations that might be instructive.

Secondly, the client's case needs to be assessed relative to the types of health complications that tend to occur in diabetics. **Atherosclerosis** is common and forms in various of parts of the arterial system, including the renal arteries; the smaller blood vessels become substantially damaged and much less responsive to temperature stimuli (**peripheral vascular disease**); **hypertension** is common and some degree of **congestive heart failure** is likely to develop; various types of **kidney disease** may occur; **sensory impairment** in the extremities is common; circulation to the skin and other surface tissues becomes compromised, making them less healthy and resilient; and immunity is compromised. Such complications tend to develop over time, and do not all always occur, so there are many variations in their presence and severity in each case. Temperature therapy is contraindicated for people with severe advanced or unstable diabetes mellitus.

- **Dyspnea**

The term dyspnea means shortness of breath, or difficulty with breathing mechanics or with gaseous exchange in the lungs. Dyspnea is not a disease in itself – it is a primary respiratory symptom and is present in a variety of respiratory conditions. Individuals with dyspnea do not have good tolerance of stimuli that increase breathing demand, such as large scale heat. Depending on the cause of their symptoms, people with dyspnea are also often unable to handle steam treatments.

- Eczema

Eczema is a superficial *dermatitis* (skin inflammation), generally of unknown cause. Sudden temperature changes, particularly heat, can exacerbate the symptoms of eczema. Eczema is a local contraindication for thermotherapy, and cryotherapy applications should be carefully monitored.

- Emphysema

Emphysema is a respiratory condition involving widespread destruction of gaseous exchange surfaces in the lungs. It is most commonly caused by long-term smoking. Emphysema is characterized by **dyspnea** – in more severe cases individuals use prescribed oxygen. Emphysema also places a great deal of stress on the heart and causes some degree of **congestive heart failure** in all sufferers. With severe emphysema the corresponding CHF is usually also severe. The long-term reduction in oxygen availability also causes poor tissue health, especially in the extremities. Each of these aspects of emphysema must be considered and matched with appropriate temperature therapy adaptations – in severe cases many applications will be too intense.

- Epilepsy

Epilepsy is characterized by *seizures*, which are the result of abnormal bursts of conduction in the brain. There are many causes and types of epilepsy – it is not a distinct disease, but rather a generic term for seizure disorder. Some seizure types are very mild and essentially harmless while others are quite dangerous and very stressful on the body, particularly the heart. People with epilepsy tend to have their specific individual seizure triggers. While many common triggers are unrelated to temperature therapy, some are directly applicable: hot or cold stimuli, sudden temperature change, water immersion (a common trigger in children), and reactions to aromas.

It is important for the temperature therapist to take a thorough case history that includes information about regular temperature practices and tolerances and any history of seizure occurrences with past temperature therapy or similar situations, for example, hot showers/baths at home or activities like swimming. Epileptic clients are also often taking medications that have numerous side effects and that may affect their ability to provide optimal feedback on how a treatment feels. Medication stability may also be a factor. With severe or unstable epileptics, or those with directly applicable triggers, some or all types of temperature therapy are likely to be contraindicated.

- Fasting

Fasting is abstention from eating. It is important to carefully monitor people who are fasting, as they may become weak and easily fatigued, states that can be aggravated by temperature therapy treatments.

- Fever

Fever is an abnormally high body temperature produced when the body fights bacterial or viral invaders. Thermotherapy applications should generally be avoided, as they may increase the fever beyond a healthy level. Cryotherapy can be effective in helping reduce fever, but should be used with caution since fever has an important purpose. When the body is fevered there is a larger temperature difference between the cryoagent and the target tissue, so cold applications should be modified toward cool.

- Frostbite

Frostbite is the result of extreme cold on the skin and subcutaneous tissues, which causes a local lack of oxygen and ultimately tissue necrosis (cell death). Cold is an absolute contraindication; heat may be used with care, utilizing warm rather than hot temperatures, but only after the frostbite has been evaluated and treated medically.

- Gangrene

Gangrene is a type of tissue death caused by loss of viable blood supply, sometimes in association with factors such as infection or inability to heal an injury. It is a serious potential complication of **peripheral vascular diseases** such as **Buerger's Disease** and **diabetes**. Pre-gangrenous states require extreme caution (with medical consultation) in using temperature therapy. Gangrene is an absolute local contraindication.

- Headaches - Vascular

Local heat should be avoided with headaches caused by increased blood flow to the head, as in a 'pounding' headache. Thermotherapy will increase the circulation and aggravate the headache.

- Hemorrhage (see Bleeding/Hemorrhage)

- Hypertension

Hypertension is chronically elevated blood pressure. It has numerous known causes (several mentioned in this list) and some that are not well understood. High blood pressure stresses the heart and over time tends to produce **congestive heart failure** – it is also implicated in **kidney disease** and stroke. Hypertension levels vary a great deal on the mild-moderate-severe continuum, and many individuals are well controlled by medication. It is important to be clear about the specific case in order to make good temperature therapy decisions.

High blood pressure is a major temperature therapy consideration, especially with full body treatments. Although heat will tend to reduce blood pressure over the course of a treatment, as discussed in Chapter 3, a full body heat application will substantially increase blood flow and venous return before the occurrence of the peripheral vasodilation that lowers pressure in the core circulation. This means that the body with hypertension, particularly if the heart is weakened, can be overtaxed in the initial response. With mild, well-controlled hypertension this effect is usually well tolerated. Full body heat treatments are not recommended for moderate hypertension, and unstable or severe hypertension is a contraindication for all but the mildest forms of temperature therapy. Be sure to check on whether the person's doctor has placed restrictions on temperature exposures.

- Hypotension

Low blood pressure raises fewer temperature therapy concerns than **hypertension**, but it is important to note that individuals with hypotension are more likely than normotensive clients to become light-headed or feel faint with intense temperature therapy applications such as steams, full body treatments, or prolonged applications.

- ## Infection

Thermotherapy is not recommended in the vicinity of an active infection because of the increase in circulation that results. This enhances the possibility of spreading the infection, either locally or more broadly.

- ## Inflammatory Bowel Disease (IBD)

Inflammatory bowel diseases include conditions such as *ulcerative colitis* and *Crohn's Disease* (*ileitis*). These are chronic, episodic, inflammatory disorders of the intestines. The reflex effects of temperature therapy must be well understood in order not to irritate or adversely affect the disordered bowel function.

- ## Kidney Disease

The kidneys, as primary organs of filtration and elimination, are responsible for continuously filtering the body's circulating blood. This role is crucial to controlling body fluid volume and toxicity levels. There are numerous causes and types of kidney disease, but common characteristics of long term conditions include progressive decline in tissue and organ system health, generalized toxicity, **hypertension** and **congestive heart failure**, and severe generalized edema. Diseased kidneys can be overstressed by treatments that mobilize large amounts of blood flow and blood pressure may spike as a result. It is important to assess the severity of each case and modify/avoid temperature therapy applications accordingly – seek medical advice as needed and proceed cautiously. Severe kidney disease is an absolute temperature therapy contraindication. Individuals receiving dialysis treatments should have medical approval before receiving temperature therapy.

- ## Liver Disease

The liver, like the kidneys, is a primary filtering and eliminatory organ, processing blood from the spleen and digestive organs before returning it to the core circulation. The concerns about temperature therapy and liver disease are essentially the same as those outlined above for **kidney disease**.

• Malignancy

Malignancy is the term used to describe cancerous growths. On-site thermotherapy is strongly discouraged because of the resulting local increase in tissue metabolism, which is thought to potentially enhance the growth and metastasis of the tumour.

• Multiple Sclerosis (MS)

Multiple sclerosis is an autoimmune disorder that affects the central nervous system in a random and widespread fashion. Each individual case is different, but there are a number of more common symptoms that influence temperature therapy treatment planning. For instance, most (not all) people with MS are very intolerant of heat and are adversely affected by heat exposures. As well, many have **sensory impairment**, abnormal sensory and reflex responses, severe fatigue, **spasticity** and other motor disorders, autonomic nervous system control problems, and *vertigo*. Vertigo, which is similar to dizziness, can be exacerbated by large scale or more intense forms of temperature therapy. Cold can be used beneficially with multiple sclerosis to reduce symptom intensity and improve energy. It is important to take careful note of the specific impairments in each client's case, but as a general rule thermotherapy is avoided and cryotherapy is used in more brief applications to avoid overstimulation. Cold may also aggravate *spasticity*.

• Neuritis

Neuritis is the inflammation of a nerve. It is very painful, and may create either reduced sensation or heightened sensitivity in the tissue the nerve supplies. Similarly, muscle tone may be low or quite spasmodic, and reflexes can be either sluggish or overly reactive. Heat is never used with inflammation. Extreme cold may also not be well tolerated, but moderated cold applications are often beneficial in helping control pain and inflammation.

154

- **Peripheral Vascular Disease (PVD)**

Peripheral vascular disease is a general term for any condition that adversely affects the function of the blood and/or lymphatic vessels, especially in the extremities. Blood flow is generally abnormal in the affected tissues, resulting in ischemia (inadequate blood supply) and paleness/cyanosis, or alternatively, congestion and edema. Signs and symptoms may also include numbness, pain, and elevated blood pressure. There may be inflammation or other symptoms specific to the cause of the condition. There can be a variety of origins of PVD, so it is important to understand the client's underlying cause(s) in order to appropriately assess which, if any, temperature therapy treatments are indicated, contraindicated, or in need of modification. Generally, circulation should not be increased through affected tissue areas, necessitating the contraindication of local and distal heat applications.

- **Phlebitis (see Arteritis/Phlebitis)**

- **Pitted Edema**

Pitted, or pitting, edema is stagnant swelling that has become less liquid and more gel-like. A depression caused by pressing the tissue with a finger remains for a time rather than rebounding immediately when released. Mild cases may respond well to moderated heat or contrast applications, assuming liquification and drainage are fairly readily achievable; otherwise local temperature therapy is not indicated because of the underlying vascular impairment.

- **Pregnancy**

Pregnancy is not a pathology and should not be over-pathologized. However, there are risks to the fetus associated with prolonged overheating of the mother's body, and temperature therapy exposures should be adjusted accordingly. In cases of high risk pregnancy, the therapist should exercise caution and take note of any restrictions placed on temperature exposures by the woman's physician.

- **Radiation Therapy**

Radiation therapy is the use of ionizing radiation in cancer treatment. The effect of the radiation is to kill cells or make them unable to reproduce. Since radiation therapy cannot be targeted to the cancer cells only, it has effects on the local normal tissues as well. Similar to sunburn, radiation treatments create burn injuries in the skin and underlying tissues that develop over a 24-48 hour period. During this time on-site water exposures are often forbidden because they can exacerbate the burn process. On-site heat would also be contraindicated. If **blisters** develop, it is best not to wet them or risk infection of the affected skin.

Any history of radiation therapy should be looked at carefully by the temperature therapist. The affected skin may remain sensitive to temperature extremes for some time. There may also be **sensory impairment** that is permanent, or that improves very slowly over time.

- **Raynaud's Disease**

Raynaud's Disease is an idiopathic condition characterized by intermittent attacks of ischemia in the extremities, particularly in the hands and fingers. This condition's symptoms can include blanching, *cyanosis* (blue colouring), numbness, tingling, burning, and pain. Cold is one of the common attack triggers and is contraindicated for use on the affected tissues. In general, the person should also avoid becoming overchilled.

- **Raynaud's Phenomenon**

Raynaud's Phenomenon involves the same signs and symptoms as Raynaud's Disease, but it is typically more severe and can include **thrombosis** risk. Raynaud's Phenomenon is so-called when it occurs secondary to another condition such as lupus.

- **Sensory Impairment**

The term sensory impairment is a generic one referring to altered sensation. The problem could originate in the CNS or PNS. While instances of heightened/excessive sensation, or abnormal sensations such as *paresthesias*, are included in the concept of sensory impairment, the term is typically used to mean sensation that is less than normal (*hypaesthesia*) or lost (*anaesthesia*). Sensation is an important aspect of temperature therapy treatment, since there is a greater risk of tissue damage when the person cannot discriminate temperature perception. Reduced or lost tissue sensation does not preclude temperature therapy use, assuming no **vasomotor impairment**, but the practitioner must be especially observant of the tissue responses. It is best to proceed with great care, using patch testing (see Chapter 5) and introducing more intense applications slowly and cautiously.

- **Spasticity**

Spasticity is a motor dysfunction that results from CNS injuries and disorders. It is characterized by reflex control problems, including poor modulation of basic protective reflexes like the muscle spindle and withdrawal reflexes, which tend to be highly reactive. Extremes of temperature are likely to precipitate spastic reactions, especially if applied suddenly. Warm applications are usually well tolerated and beneficial, but even modified cryotherapy is often problematic.

- **Superficial Pins, Wires, Rods**

Metal pins, wires, and rods are used to mend and stabilize bony structures in the body. If these appliances are exposed to extremes of heat or cold, especially heat, the metal (which is an excellent temperature conductor) can cause damage to neighbouring tissues.

- **Thrombus, Thrombosis, Deep Vein Thrombosis (DVT), Thrombophlebitis**

A *thrombus* is similar to a blood clot. Thrombosis refers to the process of thrombus development, which occurs as a result of platelet activation. Thrombosis risk is high in any situation where a blood vessel is damaged, irritated/inflamed, or has a narrowed section (*stenosis*). Extensive thrombus formation may occlude the vessel, as often happens in heart attacks. Thrombi tend to be attached to the blood vessel wall, but often loosely, so they may also break away and occlude a downstream vessel. In either case, tissue death will result. *Deep vein thrombosis* is the presence of a thrombus in a deep vein, most frequently in the leg; *thrombophlebitis* refers to an inflamed vein with thrombosis. The temperature therapist must be concerned about situations where there is an identifiable risk of exacerbating thrombosis or causing a thrombus to dislodge. Any temperature therapy applications are contraindicated that would result in increased blood flow through the affected vessel. Medical consultation is often necessary to assess safety.

- ## Transient Ischemic Attack (TIA)

Similar to what occurs in **angina pectoris**, transient ischemic attacks are the result of partially occluded arteries in the brain, usually caused by **atherosclerosis**. In circumstances where the tissue supplied by the affected artery requires more blood than the compromised blood vessel can deliver, symptoms appear. These symptoms could be any number of neurological indicators depending on the function of the affected part of the brain, for example, weakness or sensory loss on one side of the body, slurred speech, altered vision, and so on. Since these symptoms come and go, they can be overlooked, but TIAs are often stroke precursors and should be investigated and treated medically as soon as possible. When a client has diagnosed TIAs, temperature therapy is inadvisable except for mild local applications that do not generate increased systemic blood flow.

- ## Unwilling Client

Regardless of how strongly indicated or potentially beneficial you believe a temperature therapy treatment to be, if the individual is unwilling because of the temperature, the nature of the application, or any other reason, consent is not present and the treatment cannot be done.

- ## Varicose Veins - Severe

A varicose vein is a vein in which the valves that prevent backflow are incompetent – it becomes progressively more blocked, tortuous and dilated.

The most commonly affected veins are the superficial saphenous veins of the legs. Hemorrhoids are also varicosities. Older varicose veins may become weak, so in advanced cases local temperature therapy should be avoided or substantially modified.

- **Vasomotor Impairment (Paralysis or Paresis)**

The autonomic nervous system (sympathetic division) is responsible for vasoconstriction of blood vessels in the body, and for vasodilation, which is a relative absence of constriction. When there is vasomotor impairment, it can stem from problems in the control areas in the CNS, or from damage to peripheral nerves carrying the sympathetic fibres for this function. *Vasomotor paresis* is poor tone in the blood vessels due to reduced transmission; *vasomotor paralysis*, which tends to occur only from complete loss of a peripheral nerve's transmission, is full loss of vasoconstriction. When vasoconstriction is impaired blood pools in affected capillary beds – the result is a large volume of edema. When there is sluggish vasomotor function, temperature therapy must be modified in intensity to suit the available function. When there is vasomotor paralysis, local temperature therapy is to be avoided because the expected vascular reactions will not occur, eliminating the effectiveness of the applications and risking increased congestion and edema.

Now that we have discussed contraindications and cautions associated with temperature therapy decision-making, we will proceed in the next two chapters to look at what is involved in preparing for and implementing a number of specific thermotherapy, cryotherapy and contrast applications in clinical practice.

Sister Elizabeth Kenny (1886-1952) of Australia treated polio with strips of wool soaked in hot water to relieve muscle pain and to increase range of motion. Elsewhere in the world people were using braces and casts to immobilize limbs, but Kenny's treatment helped mobilize polio sufferers.

Chapter Seven

Commonly Used Treatments

Learning Objectives

After learning the contents of this chapter, the reader should be able to:

- demonstrate an understanding of appropriate uses for the treatments
- list the necessary equipment for each application
- explain the appropriate procedure for each treatment
- incorporate these treatments into clinical practice and home care recommendations

Treatments   Page

Chapter 7: Commonly Used Treatments

The specific temperature therapy treatments described in this book are divided into two groups. The first group includes commonly used applications that are accessible to most therapists for use in clinical practice and as self care, and to most clients as home care. This group also includes treatments that tend to be partial body applications or that would be considered less intense and more universally applicable, given compliance with individual contraindications. The second group involves larger scale, more intense hydrotherapy treatments. The first group is presented in this chapter and the second in Chapter 8. Some of the treatments in both chapters mention the option of incorporating additives – additives are discussed in Chapter 9.

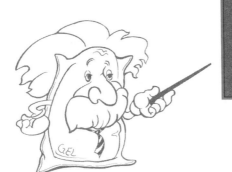

keep in mind:
The sensations caused by very cold applications are generally 'C-BAN' – cold, burning, aching numbness.

Gel Packs and Ice Bags

Gel packs and ice bags are simple to use, mould well to most target areas, and are easy applications for people to use at home. These cryotherapy treatments are helpful for acutely inflamed soft tissue conditions (e.g., bursitis, flare-up of a condition such as rheumatoid arthritis) and recent injuries (e.g., muscle strains, joint sprains).

Equipment:

- gel packs
- towels to cover gel pack or ice
- ice chips/cubes and plastic bag

Note:
Keep gel packs in the freezer ready for use – they need to be frozen for a minimum of 1 hour to be effective.

Procedure:

- Make the client comfortable and relaxed, with the target area elevated if swelling is present. Make sure the part to be treated is well supported.

- Prepare the client for what sensations to expect during the treatment: cold often burns for a short time, then aches, then feels numb (C-BAN).

- Cover the target area with a terry cloth towel. To increase the effects of the cryotherapy, wet the towel with cold water (wring out well).

- Prepare the ice cubes, ice chips, or gel pack, or use a bag with one part water and three parts chipped ice with its opening securely closed and any extra air removed. Fold the chosen application in the wet towel and place on the target tissue.

- Gently mould the pack around the contour of the body part so there is firm and even contact with the skin. Cover with a dry towel.

- Leave the pack on for no more than 10-20 minutes at a time.

- For repetitions, allow the tissue to warm to normal on its own before repeating the application.

- Feel the treated tissue area for coldness and watch for signs of frostnip.

Figure 7.1: Gel packs.

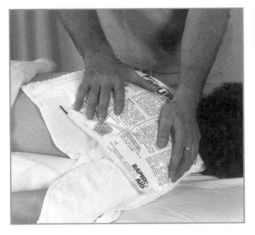 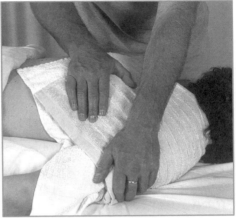

a: Contour the gel pack to
    the target tissue.

b: Cover the application
    with a towel.

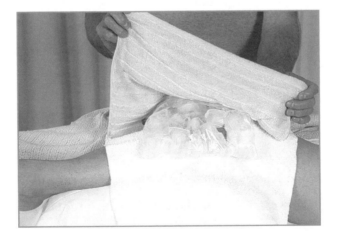

Figure 7.2: Ice bags.

Ice Massage

These cryotherapy applications are more aggressive than gel packs and ice bags. They are particularly useful for treating very localized pain and inflammation (e.g., acute ligament or tendon injuries), and after friction therapy to control any inflammation caused in the treated tissues.

Equipment:

- ice cube with popsicle stick handle or a small paper cup filled with water and frozen – the paper of the cup is peeled away to expose the ice
- towels

Procedure:

- Make the client comfortable and relaxed, with the target area elevated if swelling is present. Make sure the part to be treated is well supported.

- Test for a negative reaction to ice by putting a small piece on pre-oiled skin in a similar or adjacent tissue location to the one to be treated. After 5 minutes examine the skin for any abnormal reactions.

- Apply a small amount of oil or lotion to the tissue to be iced so the ice does not stick to and damage the skin.

- Tell the client how the ice treatment will feel: after the initial sensation of cold, there is usually a burning sensation, then an ache, and then numbness (C-BAN).

- If needed for your own comfort, wrap a small cloth or paper towel around the application so that the ice is exposed at one end.

- Make rapid movements with the ice over the target tissue, wiping drips as they develop.

- Continue the application until the treatment area feels numb to the client and cold to your touch and until the skin turns red – these results usually take several minutes.

- Be watchful for any negative reactions, such as blotching of the skin.

- Cover the treated skin when finished so it will warm up on its own.

- With deep specific techniques such as frictions, ice is used to control the inflammatory response and is standard procedure following deep tissue work.

- Brief icing can be used intermittently during some types of deeper treatments as well.

Figure 7.3: Ice massage options.

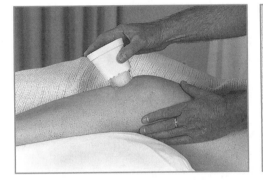

a: Ice in a paper or styrofoam cup.

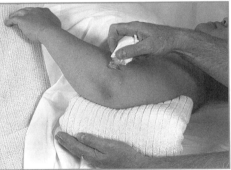

b: Ice cube held in a cloth or paper towel.

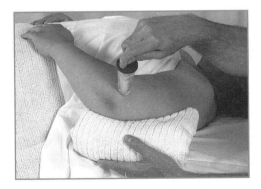

c: Popsicle stick.

Ice Bandage

By combining compression with cold, an ice bandage helps to effectively address acute inflammation at the time of an injury. These bandages should not be relied on to provide adequate immobilization, but they do serve as an effective reminder not to overuse an injured area. The wrapping should be snug, but not overly tight.

Equipment:

• dry towel or elastic bandage

• ice water

• sealed bag containing ice (ice is most effective because ice stays cold longest), or a cold gel pack.

Procedure:

• Wet an elastic bandage or long, thin towel in ice water.

• Start wrapping inferior to the injury site, and work up towards it.

• Place the ice bag over the injured tissue.

• Continue wrapping over the ice bag, holding it in place with the towel/bandage.

• Keep the ice on until swelling has noticeably diminished.

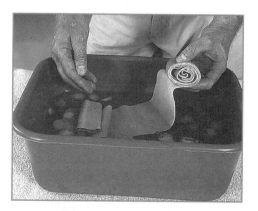

Figure 7.4: Wet the bandage in ice water.

• If continuing to use an ice bandage as a cryotherapy treatment in the days following the injury, rather than one continuous application it is now better to apply cold for 10-20 minutes, remove and let the tissue warm naturally, then re-apply.

Figure 7.5: Ice bandage.

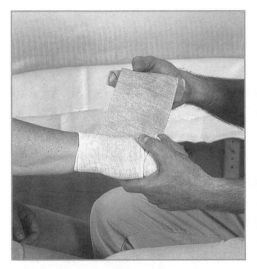

a: Wrap the wet bandage, starting inferior to the injury.

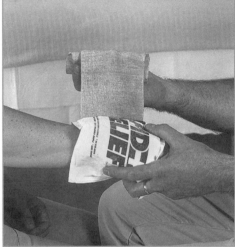

b: Once partially wrapped, apply cold gel pack.

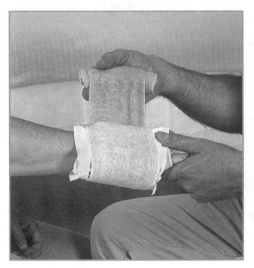

c: Continue wrapping around gel pack.

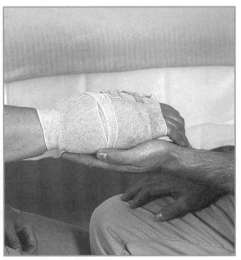

d: Finish wrapping and secure bandage clips.

Compresses and Fomentations

Compresses are folded layers of natural fibre cloths (cotton, linen, flannel) used with cold or hot water. When using hot water, compresses are called *fomentations*. Compresses mould easily to the body part being treated and are simple, effective treatments for clinic and self-care use. They have milder local effects than many other cryo- or thermoagents and can usually be tolerated for longer time periods – they are good choices for any condition where moderated heating or cooling is desired, including as a preliminary to other therapies. Compresses are a good means of modifying treatment intensity for older or more debilitated individuals, or where there is dystrophic tissue.

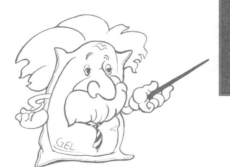

Compresses are good choices for any condition where moderated heating or cooling is desired, and as a preliminary to other therapies.

• Cold Compresses

Cold compresses are effective as a headache treatment when used on the back of the neck or on the forehead (ideally in conjunction with a hot foot bath). They can be used with any other heat modality, e.g. sauna, steam, thermophore to help avoid overheating or vasodilation-induced headache. They are helpful after a heat treatment, such as a hydrocollator pack, to restore tone to the skin and help reduce any excessive local fluid accumulation. They are also easily adapted for home use.

Cold compresses are made of natural fibre cloth that is well wrung out in cold water and applied directly to the skin. For greater intensity, ice water can be used. They are *not* covered with a dry towel. The cloth is changed regularly either by being re-folded to expose inner layers that are still cold, or by being replaced with another well wrung out cloth. The compress has to be kept cold to maintain the vasoconstrictive (retrostatic) effect on the skin – otherwise it will function as a heating compress (discussed below). Cold compresses are best used in a series, so have on hand 1 or 2 additional towels that can be applied when the one on the body warms up.

Cold compresses are also often chosen in situations where the goal is to achieve reflex effects in organs. They can be placed directly onto the skin reflex area (see Figure 1.10 in Chapter 1) for the structure to be treated (e.g., the liver, intestines).

Remember to avoid chilling the client, particularly when cold compresses are used after a hot treatment.

Equipment:

- cold water (1°C/34°F)
- small bucket
- 2-3 small towels

171

Procedure:

- Make sure that the room is not cool or drafty.

- Wring out the cloth well.

- Place the compress over the body part to be treated – do not cover the cloth.

- Re-apply a fresh cold compress or re-fold the cloth as soon as the application no longer feels cold to the client (avoid the vasodilation of derivation).

- Remove the compress and cover the skin or dry it off.

Figure 7.6: Cold compress.

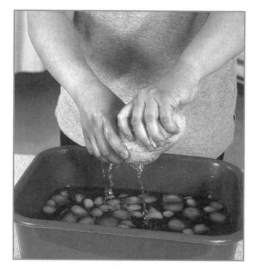
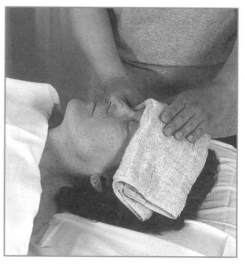

a: Wet the towel in ice water and wring out well.

b: Apply to the target tissue with no covering.

• Fomentations

The application of a series of hot, moist towels is helpful for chronic soft tissues conditions, particularly when the weight of a hydrocollator cannot be tolerated. Fomentations are sometimes called *alternating hot towels*. Sore muscles and stiff joints are often helped by the moist heat of hot towels. This application is also easily employed for home care. Fomentations are covered with a dry cloth or towel to help sustain the heat.

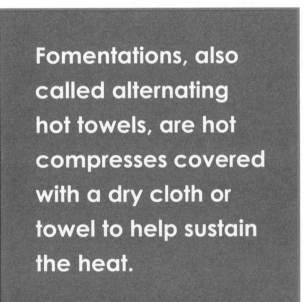

Fomentations, also called alternating hot towels, are hot compresses covered with a dry cloth or towel to help sustain the heat.

Equipment:

- 2-3 towels (thicker towels retain heat better)
- 1 dry towel for covering the application area
- rubber gloves (optional)
- bucket
- kettle or other heat source
- hot water (approximately 40°C/104°F); can be modified for a warm versus hot fomentation

Procedure:

- Have the hot water ready.
- Fold the towels to fit the tissue area being treated.
- Dip the towel in the water, leaving the ends out to facilitate wringing.
- Place the hot towel on the skin. Initially, you should quickly lift the towel off a few times to allow the skin to adjust to the heat and to prevent burning with hotter applications.
- Cover the treated area with a dry towel.
- If necessary, apply a cold compress to the neck or forehead to prevent overheating.
- When the towel begins to cool (after 3-5 minutes), place a second hot, wrung out towel on top, then flip the whole set of towels over and remove the old towel. This procedure keeps the skin from chilling between towels.
- Repeat as required. The treatment usually lasts for 10-30 minutes, but may be shorter if it is being used as a preliminary to other therapies.
- You can wipe the treated part with a cool cloth afterwards.

Figure 7.7: Fomentations.

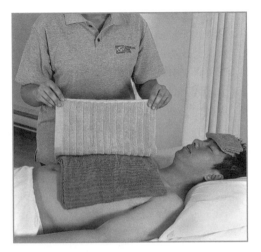

a: Apply hot compress covered by thinner dry towel.

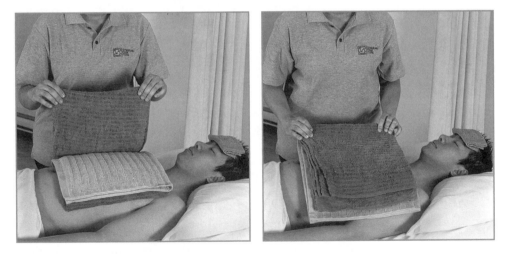

b: To replace first hot towel, cover fomentation with new hot towel.

c: Flip over entire application, then remove old towel from the top.

175

• Hot Towel Roll

A hot towel roll uses hot towels that do not need replenishing because the entire roll is heated and the cooled outer layers of towel are gradually removed. Hot towel rolls are helpful for chronic soft tissue conditions such as a sprain or strain that is nearly resolved. They can also be employed, adding more light friction with the towel roll, to help desquamate and stimulate the skin (for instance, after cast removal).

Equipment:

- 3-4 towels (not too thick); inner layer can be linen

- kettle

- water

Procedure:

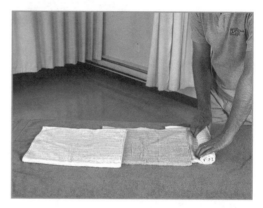

Figure 7.8: Roll the towels in a staggered formation to create a funnel at the roll's centre.

- Lay the first towel down and begin rolling it up very tightly: the length depends on the size of the tissue being covered, but the towel should be small enough to roll easily.

- Leave 15 cm (6") at the end and add the second towel; if the towels are folded, leave the folded edge approximately 5 cm (2") over the other folded edge so that it will protrude when the roll is done.

- Continue in the same manner with the third and fourth towels.

- You should ultimately have a manageable roll with 1 end indented and the folded edges protruding in a funnel-like arrangement.

- *Slowly* pour approximately 1 litre (1/4 gallon) of boiling water into the centre of the roll until you feel the warmth reach the outside towel.

- Massage the body part with the towel roll, then roll the towels one at a time onto the skin and roll off the cooling outer towels.

Figure 7.9: Hot towel roll treatment.

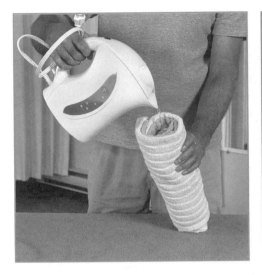

a: Pour boiling water into the centre of the towel roll.

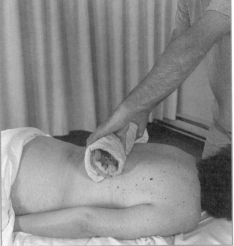

b: Massage the target area with the hot roll.

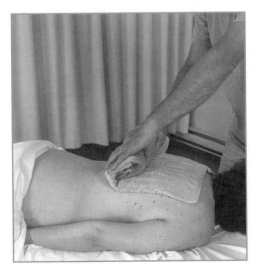

c: As the outer towel cools, unroll it onto the body part.

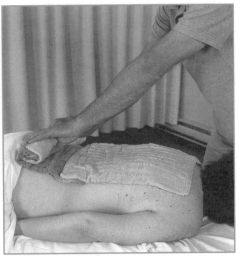

d: Remove outer towel and resume.

• Contrast Towels

This treatment is the application of a series of hot and cold towels to a specific tissue to induce vascular flushing.

Contrast towels are helpful for stimulating local circulation and drainage. They are especially effective for tissues that are healing and cannot yet handle heavy applications, such as joint sprains, muscle strains and post-surgical conditions that have started to resolve and are in the sub-acute or early chronic stage of inflammation. Any contraindications to heat are applicable to contrast towels.

Procedure:

- Use the same method as for fomentations (above), beginning with hot towels and following with cold towels.

- The usual duration of the applications is 1-3 minutes for the hot (these towels tend to lose their heat fairly quickly, especially as they are applied to cooled skin) and 30-60 seconds for the cold.

- Repeat the process at least 3 times.

- Alternative heat:cold patterns may be used, as discussed in Chapter 4.

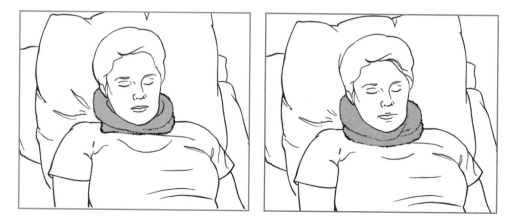

Figure 7.10: Contrast towels.

• Contrast Head Compresses

This treatment involves the use of contrast temperature compresses on the head, face, or neck. Contrast head treatments are very helpful in addressing congestion from colds, sinus problems, and from tension due to stress. They can also be helpful for skin conditions such as acne. The effects of contrast head compresses can be enhanced with a simultaneous warm foot bath.

Equipment:

*   two basins, or a gel pack and a thermophore (hydrocollator pack may be too heavy)
*   hot water (about 40°C/104°F)
*   cold water (1°C/34°F)
*   several small towels

Procedure:

*   Apply a hot compress to the head for 3-5 minutes.
*   Place a cold compress (a gel pack can be included) to the head for no longer than 1 minute.
*   Repeat the procedure 3-5 times.
*   It is generally best to finish with a cold application.

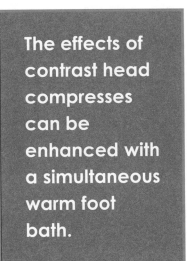

The effects of contrast head compresses can be enhanced with a simultaneous warm foot bath.

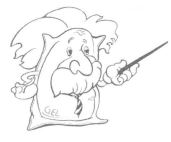

• Contrast Chest Compresses

These treatments involve the use of contrast temperature compresses to the chest. Contrast chest treatments are helpful with respiratory congestion, lactation problems, and tender, congested breasts.

Equipment:

- two basins, or a gel pack and a thermophore (hydrocollator pack may be too heavy)
- hot water (about 40°C/104°F)
- cold water (1°C/34°F)
- several small towels

Procedure:

- Place a fomentation over the chest for 3-5 minutes.
- Apply a cold compress for less than 1 minute.
- Repeat the applications 4-6 times.
- Generally end the treatment with cold.
- Dry the chest immediately, and make sure the person warms up completely (under a blanket if necessary).

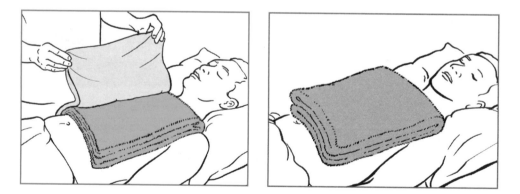

Figure 7.11: Contrast chest compresses.

- **Heating Compress**

Heating compresses use *cold* water. They are left on until the secondary action of derivation occurs and blood flows back to the treated surface tissue to warm it up. Remember that blood flow will always come from a congested area first before coming from other parts of the body. It is in utilizing this principle that heating compresses are so successful.

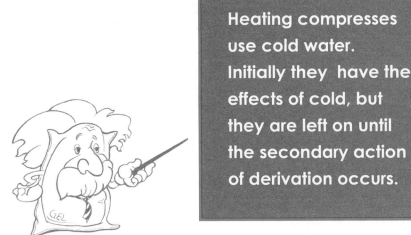

Heating compresses use cold water. Initially they have the effects of cold, but they are left on until the secondary action of derivation occurs.

These treatments help to relieve deep congestion by mobilizing circulation towards the skin surface, and help to detoxify by promoting mild local perspiration. This detoxification effect can be enhanced by adding cider vinegar to the water.

A heating compress can be described as a *cold double compress* because the cold cloth is covered with a dry one to preserve the heat that is being drawn from the body into the underlying cloth. The dry cloth keeps the warmed air trapped inside.

Heating compresses are best applied around the throat, around joints, to calf muscles, and on the abdomen (where they can be used to address insomnia and constipation). The primary goal is to relieve congestion, although there is often a sedative/relaxation effect in the treated tissues. On the neck,

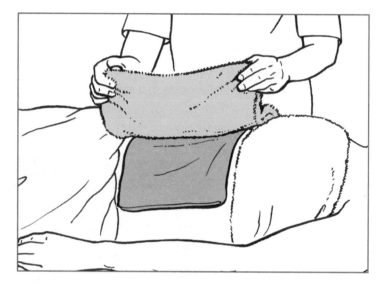

Figure 7.12: Abdominal heating compress.

heating compresses are helpful for treating sore throats and laryngitis. For earaches, a similar process can be followed, wrapping a cloth under the chin to cover the ears and securing it with a pin or knot on the top of the head.

The compress is left on until it feels warm (up to 30 minutes). To achieve a stronger effect you may decide to re-apply cold; after it warms again the compress is left on for half an hour or removed for additional treatment modalities. When employed for home care, the warmed compress can be left on for up to 2 hours or overnight.

Equipment:

- linen or cotton cloth
- pail of cold water
- 1 large towel to cover the wet compress
- vinegar to enhance the stimulus (optional)

Procedure:

- Add any additives to the water, as desired.

- Fold 1 cloth (size of folds to match the target area) and wring it out well in cold water. If the cloth is too wet the body may have to work too hard to heat it up, possibly leading to a negative reaction.

- Apply the cloth quickly to the body part and cover snugly with a dry towel.

- Leave the compress on until it feels warm. Another compress can be applied (more stimulating), or the compress can be left on for a suitable time period.

- Check with the client to make sure she or he feels the compress warming up within 10 minutes from the initial, or any repeated, application.

- If the treated tissue does not warm up, this is considered a paradox reaction and should be responded to accordingly (see Chapter 5).

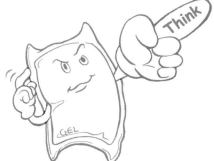

With a heating compress treatment, if the treated tissue does not warm up, this is considered a negative reaction (paradox reaction).

Foot Baths

Foot baths involve submersion of the feet and legs up to the mid-calf using warm, cold, or contrast temperatures.

• Warm Foot Bath

Warm foot baths can be used to help combat congestive headaches, to enhance the drawing of blood away from congested body areas during applications such as cold compresses or steams, and to warm up a chilled body.

Equipment:

- basin/bucket large enough for feet and deep enough for the water level to reach mid-calf
- water at 36°-38°C (96°-100°F)

Procedure:

- Have the client sit comfortably with her or his legs exposed to the knees (or the lower body undressed for better sweating).
- Add selected additive(s) to the water, e.g. Epsom salts, mustard flour (optional).
- Have the individual put her or his feet in the water.
- Cover the person with a cotton sheet or blanket for warmth or to enhance perspiration, if desired.
- Apply a cold compress to the neck if needed to prevent overheating.
- You can do a massage in the water if specifically addressing a foot concern.
- Leave the feet in for 5-20 minutes, adding hot water as needed to maintain warmth; have the client move her or his feet to the edge of the basin during the re-fill to avoid contact with the hot water.

Figure 7.13: Foot bath treatment.

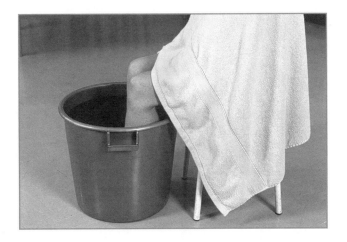

a: *Fill bucket so water level is at client's mid-calf.*

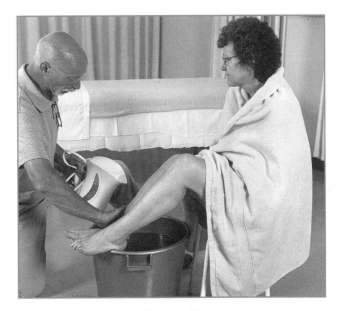

b: *When adding hot water to a warm foot bath, make sure client's legs are out of the way.*

- You can finish with a cold rinse if the purpose is to increase circulation.

- Thoroughly dry the feet and put on wool or cotton socks to avoid chilling.

• Cold Foot Bath

Cold foot baths can be used to energize tired, achy feet and legs. A cold foot bath can also be used unilaterally to address a specific problem requiring a cold foot application, for example if there are sprains to intrinsic foot joints, or to achieve contralateral effects in a casted foot/leg.

Equipment:

- large basin
- cold water: 4°-20°C (39°-68°F) – as cold as tolerable

Procedure:

- Fill the bucket with cold water.
- Submerge the client's legs and feet in the water to mid-calf depth.
- Keep in the water for 10-120 seconds or until aching is felt.
- Remove from the water and dry thoroughly.
- Put on warm socks.
- Follow up with light exercise such as walking.

• Contrast Foot Bath

A contrast foot bath uses warm and cold temperatures to cause a flushing effect and increase in local circulation. Contrast foot baths are helpful when the person has sluggish metabolism or the fatigue/lethargy associated with mild anemia or low blood pressure. These applications are commonly used for late sub-acute or chronic injuries, chronically edematous feet, mild lower limb circulation problems, and 'tired legs.'

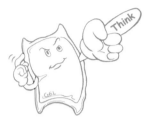

Clients should be monitored well during contrast foot baths, especially individuals who are unused to hydrotherapy treatments, since nausea can result from large temperature changes.

Equipment:

- 2 large basins
- warm (36°-38°C/97°-100°F) and cold (4°-20°C/39°-68°F) water
- cold compress
- kettle
- sheet and blanket

Procedure:

- Have the person disrobe from the knees or waist down.
- Check the pulse.
- The duration of the treatment is 3-5 minutes for warm, and 10-30 seconds for cold (or until aching is felt).
- Repeat the cycle at least 3 times beginning with warm and ending with cold.
- Alternative heat:cold patterns may be used, as discussed in Chapter 4.
- Check the person's pulse every 5 minutes, or more frequently if the person has a vascular condition or diabetes.
- After the treatment, wipe off the feet, dry thoroughly, and put on warm socks.
- People often need to rest afterward.

Tonic Friction Applications

Friction is mainly used as a stimulant and to prepare the body for cryotherapy In this context the word friction is being used differently than in manual therapy. The effects achieved depend on the intensity of the treatment. A light scratching application causes slight contraction of small surface blood vessels. A more energetic friction will cause surface vessels to contract initially, and then dilate as blood flow returns to the skin. A strong vigorous treatment will result in hyperemia of the skin and increased heat elimination. Friction also exfoliates the skin. The term *tonic* refers to the stimulation of a *strengthening reaction* – there is a resultant improvement in the skin's tone and its ability to withstand cold temperatures.

Cold mitten friction, *dry brushing*, and *salt glows* all employ friction. The therapist can use these techniques to increase the client's tolerance of more intense cold treatments. They also improve the efficiency of the skin's elimination function.

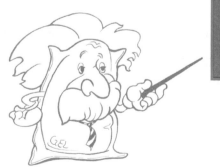

The term tonic refers to the stimulation of a strengthening reaction.

• Cold Mitten Friction

A cold mitten friction is an application of cold water to the skin with friction, using a wash mitt or small towel, to increase circulation to the skin. Such a treatment stimulates skin circulation while being much milder on the heart than other full body cold applications. This type of application is an excellent means of training the vascular system to react positively to cold, of addressing fatigue and lethargy, and of stimulating the skin after cast removal. Since cold mitten friction enhances heat escape from the skin, it can be good for reducing fevers. It can also be used to achieve visceral reflex effects associated with brief cold applications.

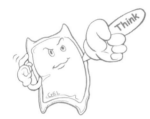

This sort of treatment should never be used over skin lesions or an open sore – the wound must be carefully avoided. It is also important to ensure that recent scar tissue is not damaged.

Equipment:

- natural fibre mitten or small towel folded around the hand
- bucket of cold water

Procedure:

- Ensure the client is warm and comfortable. This application is usually done with the person lying down.
- Dip the mitt or towel in water and wring out well.
- Uncover the target tissue and rub vigorously, using moderate pressure.
- Cover the part immediately after it receives the application to avoid chilling, but *do not dry off*. A film of water adhering to the skin induces the skin temperature to rise gradually to re-warm the area. If the person is debilitated, each body part can be friction-dried with a clean, dry towel before the next is treated.

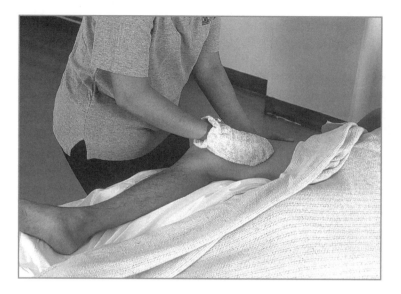

Figure 7.14: Cold mitten friction.

Application Pattern:

Supine:

- Start with the foot, then move up the shin, then treat the thigh from lateral to medial. The calf and posterior thigh can be treated in supine position with the knee bent if desired.

- Treat the other leg in the same way.

- Friction the hand and up the arm, going from lateral to medial and addressing both anterior and posterior surfaces.

- Treat the chest and abdomen, being sure to friction the abdomen in a clockwise direction.

Prone:

- Do the posterior legs if not already done.

- Treat the upper back and the lower back, including the gluteals and over the sacrum.

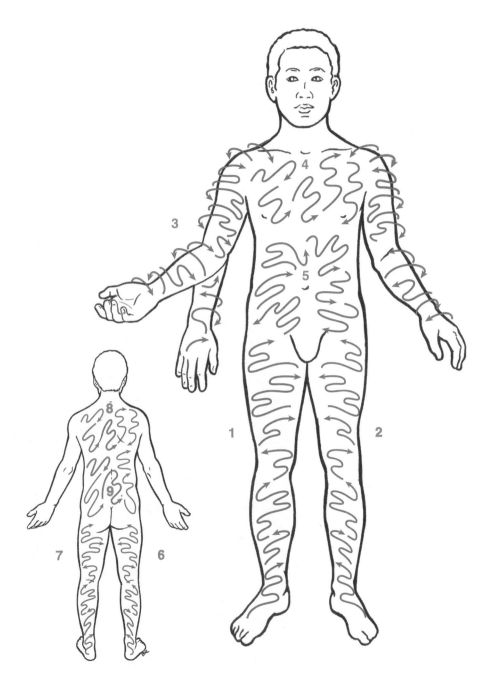

Figure 7.15: Cold mitten friction full body treatment pattern.

• Dry Brushing

Dry brushing is the use of a dry, natural fibre brush to massage the body, partially or completely, to directly stimulate the circulation of the skin.

This is a friction-based treatment that is done with brisk, circular, long movements with more obvious pressure towards the heart than cold mitten friction. Dry brushing is a stimulating treatment that is well suited to being done in the morning as an overall tonic to the body. It helps to slough off dead skin cells, making it a good choice after cast removal or for someone who is bedridden, provided that the skin is not too fragile. It is also a good treatment to help tone the skin in preparation for full body treatments, for instance prior to or during a sauna to enhance perspiration. It is important not to work on broken skin such as acne, inflamed or open lesions, or skin that has been freshly shaven. Body areas with a lot of hair may be excessively irritated by this type of treatment.

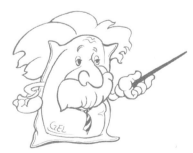

Dry brushing is a stimulating treatment that is well suited to being done in the morning as an overall tonic to the body. Areas of treatment should be changed daily to avoid acclimatizing, i.e., do upper, lower, or full body on alternating days.

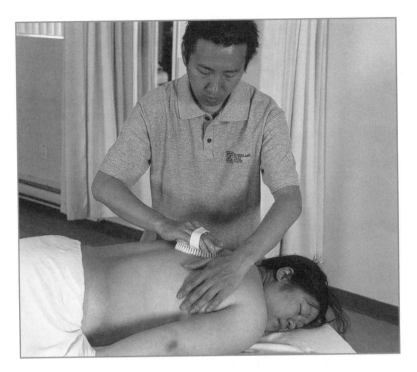

Figure 7.16: Dry brushing.

Equipment:

- natural fibre brush, bath mitten, or rough towel

Procedure:

- This treatment can be done with the client lying down or standing up.

- The brush is always used dry, not moistened.

- The direction of pressure is toward the heart.

- Areas of treatment should be changed daily to avoid acclimatizing, i.e., do upper, lower, *or* full body on alternating days.

- The full body treatment should last 5 minutes maximum, or until hyperemia results. Hyperemia is produced more quickly in the torso, while the limbs (especially lower) might not show much redness. Stop brushing before irritation results, keeping in mind that the torso is more easily irritated than the extremities. Hyperemia appears more readily with repeated use as circulation improves.

- Brush the limbs from lateral to medial to acclimatize the tissue – the inner surfaces are more sensitive.

- If the brushing feels irritating to the person, you can follow with a soothing stroke with your other hand.

Application Pattern:

Supine:

- Use long, circular, arc-like movements.

- Start with the right foot and sole, then move to the shin, then the thigh from exterior to interior. Use less pressure in the inner thigh region. Repeat on the left leg. You can include the posterior leg or wait until the client is prone.

- Brush up the right hand and arm (exterior to interior), then the left hand and arm.

- Brush the chest toward the sternum.

- Brush the abdomen in a clockwise direction (mirror the direction of peristaltic flow).

Prone:

- Do the posterior legs if not already done.

- Brush the upper and lower back, including the gluteals and over the sacrum.

194

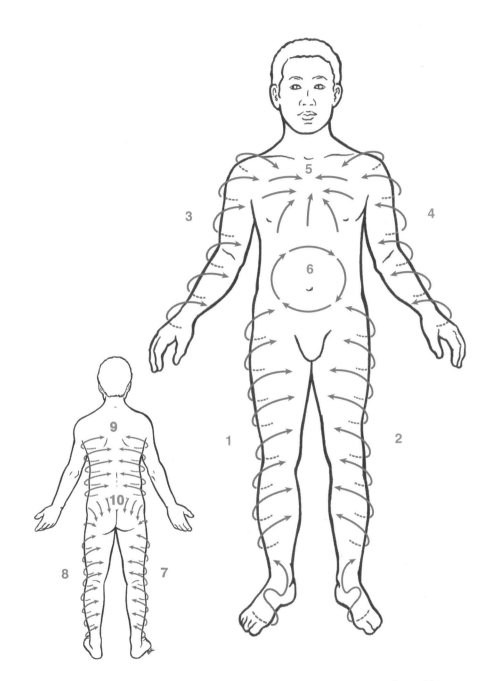

Figure 7.17: Dry brushing full body treatment pattern.

• Salt Glow

A salt glow involves the application of slightly moistened salt to the body using friction. Salt glows are excellent for increasing skin circulation and stimulating cutaneous nerves. They are very effective for removing dead cells and softening rough skin. These treatments help to gradually increase people's responsiveness to and tolerance of cold applications. If perspiration is reduced or sluggish, a salt glow is a good method of stimulating the sweat glands in preparation for a full body treatment like a sauna.

Salt glows should not be done on open wounds, including acne, or recent scar tissue. Warn clients that a salt rub on recently shaven skin will sting, so they should avoid shaving the target area(s) just prior to a treatment.

Equipment:

*   small bowl and small amount of water
*   salt: coarse, pickling, Epsom, or sea salt (some people find Epsom salt less irritating); amount depends on the size of the person; 1-2 cups
*   may use a massage table covered in a sheet or large towel, or a bath tub – as a home care option, the person can do a salt glow while standing in the tub, then run hot water for a salt bath
*   wash cloth and small bucket, or shower stall (for washing off after the treatment)

Procedure:

*   Salt glows can be done with the client lying down, standing, or seated.
*   Put in a bowl the amount of salt required to treat the target tissue(s).
*   Moisten the salt in the bowl so that the salt sticks together slightly.
*   Have the person standing comfortably on a towel or mat, or sitting on a stool in the tub, or lying on the table.
*   Place moistened salt between your hands and apply it to the body with friction in a saw-like motion.

- Modify the pressure as indicated, e.g., use deeper pressure on fleshy regions and less pressure on bony areas.

- Have the person rinse or shower with cool/cold water.

- If the treated skin shows signs of irritation, apply a mild moisturizer.

Application Pattern:

Supine:

- Begin with the legs, working from the feet to the hips.

- Treat the arms, beginning with the hands and working up to the shoulders.

- Next do the chest and abdomen, applying pressure in a clockwise direction on the abdomen.

Prone:

- Treat the back and gluteal area.

- Treat the posterior legs, working from the feet to the hips.

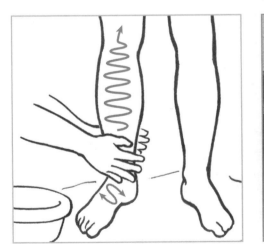 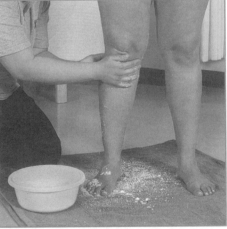

Figure 7.18a & b: Salt glows are applied with friction in a saw-like motion.

Washings

A washing involves applying, and leaving, a thin film of water on the skin. Leaving the water to evaporate from the skin surface intensifies the treatment effect. Washings can be full body, partial, or done in a series.

The temperature of the water should be cold; however, *cool* temperatures should be utilized when treating older people, young children, and clients who are unable or unwilling to tolerate cold temperature. Warm or tepid water can be used when fevers are accompanied by chills and aches.

Full body washings are considered the mildest form of all the hydrotherapy treatments. Assuming temperature modifications are made if needed, there are very few contraindications. These treatments can help to increase energy levels (especially when done first thing in the morning) and to stimulate temperature regulation. They can also be soothing, and, when used before bed, can help with insomnia or restless sleep. Full body washings can be helpful for poor circulation. Washings can also be used to help people become more tolerant of cryotherapy treatments.

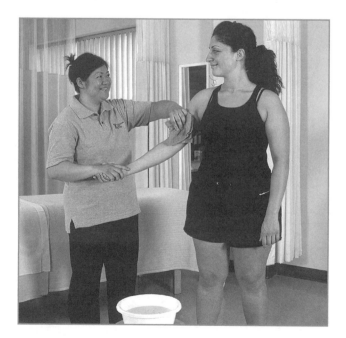

Figure 7.19: Washing.

- ## Full Body Washing

Equipment:

- linen or rough cotton cloth, approximately 30 cm x 30 cm
- bucket of cold water
- for increased stimulation, add vinegar or salt

Procedure:

The following procedure describes the full body washing routine. Partial applications would use the sections of this procedure that describe washing of the body part(s) chosen for the treatment.

- The entire full body treatment is done very quickly to avoid excessively chilling the client. It should take *less than 2 minutes*.
- Wring out the cloth well prior to the application.

Note: Wipe twice in the creases, e.g. inguinal crease, gluteal crease, axilla.

Application Pattern:

- Fold the cloth in four, securing it well in your hand.
- This treatment is often done with the client standing, but lying down is easily accommodated.
- Beginning with the client's right hand, quickly wash up the posterior aspect of the arm to the right shoulder, then return to the hand via the anterior surface, then medially up to the axilla – wipe twice.
- Turn the cloth and repeat with the client's left arm.
- Rinse the cloth.
- Wipe the right then the left side of the neck.
- Wipe in a **W** form on the chest (avoid nipple contact).
- Turn the cloth and wipe under the breasts if appropriate.

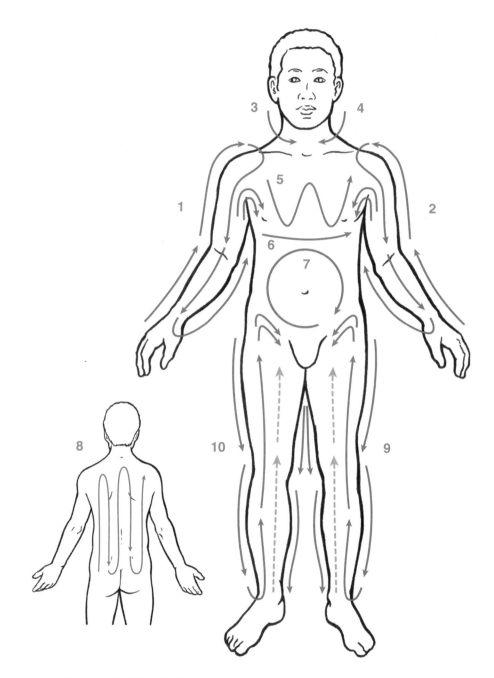

Figure 7.20: Full body washing treatment pattern.

- Rinse the cloth.

- Wipe clockwise around the abdomen.

- Rinse the cloth.

- Wipe the back and gluteals with brisk vertical movements.

- Rinse the cloth.

- Wipe one leg at a time: Wipe up the posterior aspect, down the lateral side, up the anterior aspect, wipe twice in the inguinal crease, then wipe down the medial side.

- Be sure the client rests for a while after the washing and is comfortably warm to avoid post-treatment chilling.

• Abdominal Washing

Abdominal washings are a gentle method of reflexively stimulating the intestines to ease constipation. They are also generally relaxing. Abdominal washings done in bed just before sleep as self care can help address insomnia.

Equipment:

- as for Full Body Washing

Procedure:

- Position the client supine with her or his knees flexed and supported to relax the abdominal muscles.

- Beginning on the skin above the ileocecal valve in the lower right abdominal quadrant, make clockwise motions 20-40 times.

- Refold and rinse the cloth often to keep it cool.

- Allow the client to rest and warm up afterward, using a blanket if needed.

Thermophore

Thermophores are electrical fomentation devices that create moist heat. They are available in various sizes. The thermophore's flannel cover traps moisture from the air and body surface, which creates a different, more intense effect than a dry heating pad.

Thermophores are helpful for chronic soft tissue conditions such as achy, tight muscles and for warming a chilled client by placing it on her or his back or feet. A thermophore application on the back is very relaxing. For many types of bodywork that involve treatment on a table with sheets, the thermophore is ideal for warming the sheets prior to the client's arrival. It is also commonly used to cover a paraffin-waxed area to maintain the heat of the wax treatment.

This treatment must be monitored in order to avoid burning as this type of pack produces an intense heat. *Never lay the thermophore under the client.*

Equipment:

- electric thermophore
- keep flannel clean for hygienic reasons
- thin towel

Procedure:

- Place the warmed thermophore on the thin towel over the target tissue. For more fragile clients, allow the fomentation to warm up on the client.
- Do not let the client lie on the thermophore.
- Check for hyperemia and heat sensitivity by looking at and feeling the skin under the thermophore from time to time during the treatment.
- Make sure the heat level is within the client's tolerance.
- Remove the thermophore after 20-30 minutes maximum.
- You can wipe the skin with a cool cloth afterwards.

Figure 7.21: Thermophore.

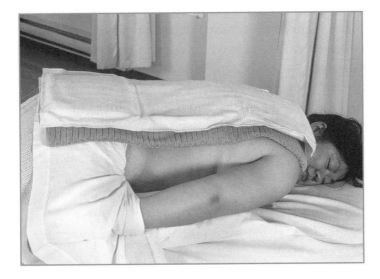

a: Always place a towel between the thermophore and the skin.

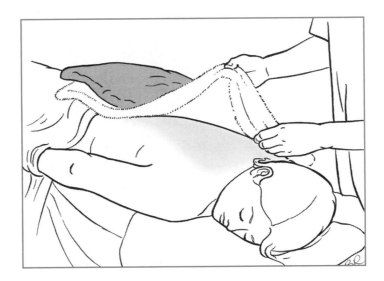

b: Check the skin under the thermophore periodicallly.

Hydrocollator

A hydrocollator pack is a silica gel filled pack that is soaked in hot water to provide prolonged moist heat. A hydrocollator pack is good in any situation that requires penetrating heat, and is an especially good choice for conditions such as hyperkyphosis that benefit from weight in addition to the heat – the larger packs are somewhat heavy when wet. For the same reason, a hydrocollator pack should not be used if the weight of the pack is excessive for the person's constitution or the tissue being treated.

New packs are dry, so soak them for one hour in tepid water, then heat them in the hydrocollator unit. For home use they can be heated in a large pot. The packs should not be allowed to dry out after use, as they tend to crack and do not re-hydrate well. Between treatments, keep hydrocollator packs covered in water in a heated hydrocollator unit, or frozen in a plastic bag. They do not keep well at room temperature.

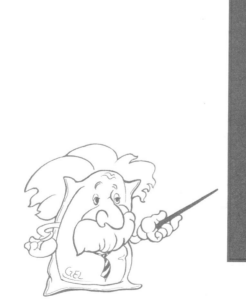

A hydrocollator pack is good in any situation that requires penetrating heat, and is an especially good choice for conditions such as hyperkyphosis that benefit from weight in addition to the heat.

Equipment:

- professional hydrocollator heating unit or deep pot
- hydrocollator moist heat pack (they are available in various shapes and sizes)
- keep water in unit refreshed and clean the unit regularly
- towels or commercial pack cover

Procedure:

- Let the pre-soaked pack warm up in hot water for a minimum of 20 minutes.

- For applying this treatment at home, bring a large pot of water to boil, then turn the element off and put the pack in, letting it heat for 20 minutes.

- Fold a towel on the tissue to be treated, making two layers.

- Wrap the gel pack in towels – 3-5 layers underneath and 1 on top, or use a commercial pack cover.

- Lay the pack on client.

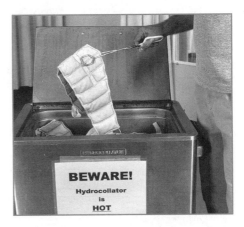

Figure 7.22: Always handle hydrocollator packs with tongs.

- If the client reports the application feels too hot, add layers of towels; if the body part does not feel warm enough, remove a layer or two.

- Heat is given off for about 30 minutes, and the effects in the tissue can continue for as much as an hour after the treatment.

- The treatment can last 10-30 minutes depending on the needs of the tissue. Check the tissue frequently.

- The skin can be wiped with a cool cloth or compress afterwards.

205

Figure 7.23: Hydrocollator packs.

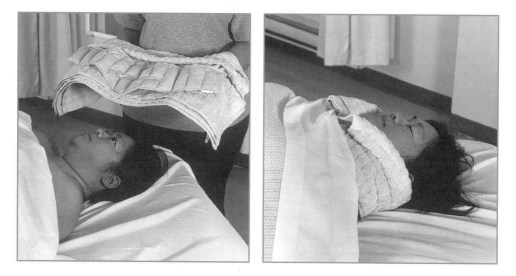

a & b: Cervical hydrocollator pack treatment.

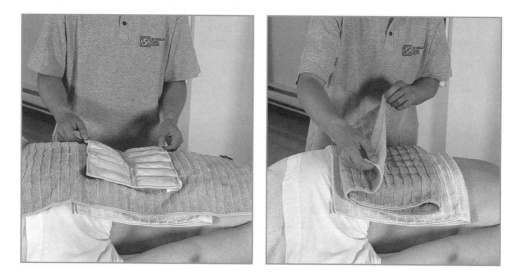

c & d: Lumbar hydrocollator pack treatment.

Paraffin Wax Bath

A paraffin wax bath involves the therapeutic application of melted paraffin wax to the target tissue to create a deep, moist heat. The paraffin creates a seal that prevents release of heated air from the skin surface. A fine layer of perspiration forms under the wax that continues to conduct heat into the tissue below the application, especially if there is thin plastic wrap and another heat source (e.g., a thermophore or hydrocollator pack) on top of the wax application.

Paraffin wax treatments are effective in addressing scar tissue and adhesions, as well as trophic changes in skin. They are also effective in addressing stiff joints when used in combination with exercise and/or massage. The heat penetrates well into connective tissue structures. *Never apply paraffin wax directly over severe varicose veins.*

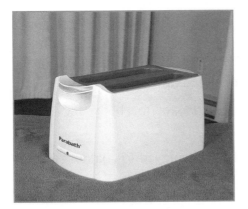

Figure 7.24: Commercial paraffin wax bath unit.

Note: Paraffin preparations for therapeutic use can be purchased pre-mixed at a medical supply store or plain paraffin can be found in grocery and hardware stores. If you get plain paraffin, it must be mixed with mineral oil at an 8-9:1 ratio (8 or 9 parts paraffin, 1 part mineral oil). The mineral oil helps to prevent cracking of the application, lowers the melting temperature of the wax, and prevents the wax from pulling out hair. Paraffin wax alone has a melting temperature of 55°C (130°F), but the therapeutic applications are applied at a temperature a few degrees lower. Wax has low thermal conductivity, which prevents burning of the skin because it emits heat more slowly than other agents.

Equipment:

- paraffin wax mixture

- commercial wax bath unit

- for home use, have a crock pot or double boiler (caution the client about possible burning from touching the edges or bottom when dipping the hands or feet into the pot)

- silicone brush

- plastic wrap

- towels

- additional heating source, e.g. thermophore (optional)

Procedure:

- Prepare the client for a possible tingling and drawing sensation initially.

- With hands, elbows, and feet, the body part is dipped. Ensure cleanliness of the treated part(s) to decrease the risk of bacterial build-up in the wax pot, particularly if not using a commercial wax bath.

- For scars, or for shoulders and other areas of the body, the wax is painted on.

- When dipping the hands, keep the fingers splayed to coat all surfaces evenly and to avoid cracking.

- Dip or paint up to 10 layers.

- The initial layer should be the highest or widest to create the initial seal with the skin.

- Wrap the area in plastic then in towels and leave for 20 minutes.

- A heat source can be added over or wrapped around the treated part to intensify the effect of the application.

- The treatment is self-insulating because the first layer traps the air: ideally you should not dip/paint the subsequent layers beyond the edge of the first layer.

- The tissue will cool quickly after wax removal. It is helpful to exercise and/or massage afterwards to prevent stiffening and to make use of the increased mobility.

- The used wax can be used as an exercise tool for the hands by manipulating it shaped as a ball.

- Never return used wax to the wax bath.

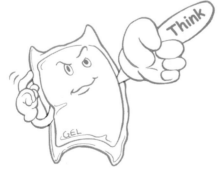

Note: **A commercial wax bath unit is self-sterilizing. When it is plugged in, it heats up to 65°C (150°F) and then cools down. Exercise caution whenever you plug in a unit as the temperature will temporarily increase to sterilizing temperature.**

Figure 7.25: Paraffin wax bath dipping.

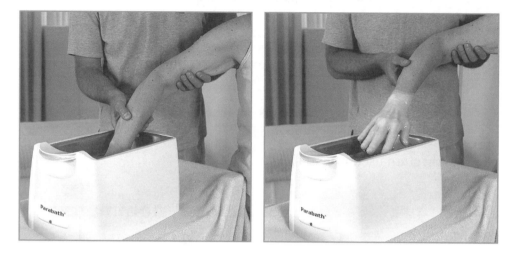

a: For dipping treatments, assist the client to ensure no contact with the unit's sides.

b: When dipping the hand, client's fingers should be splayed for even coverage.

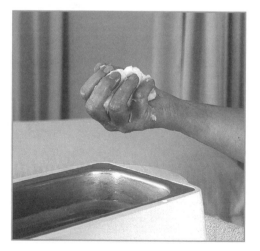

c: The used wax is a good exercise tool for the hand.

Figure 7.26: Paraffin wax painting.

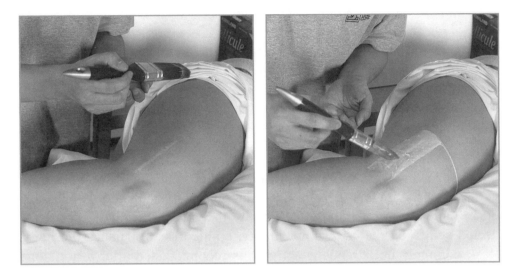

a: Paraffin painting is ideal
for scar treatments.

b: The initial layer is the
largest.

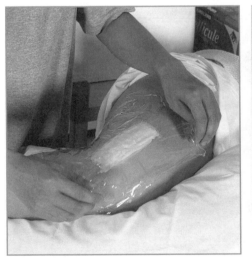

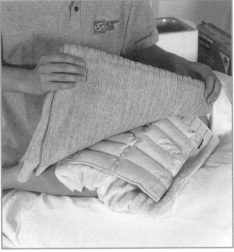

c: Paint about 10 layers, then
cover with thin plastic.

d: Cover the wax treatment
with a hydrocollator pack.

Hot Stone Massage

Hot stone massage helps enhance the effects of deep or relaxing massage by coupling heat with the massage techniques. Massaging with hot stones can also reduce strain on the therapist's hands, as not as much pressure is needed to attain tissue depth. Therapists should choose the size of the stones based on their own hand comfort and on the size of the body part being massaged. The stones should be marble or basalt (lava rock) as these are non-porous stones that retain heat especially well.

Hot stone massages are effective for inducing relaxation and for addressing muscle pain and tension. This application requires that plenty of oil be used to diminish friction on the skin. Essential oils can be added to the massage oil to increase the relaxing effect. Many therapists also place crystals or heated stones on the *chakra*, or energy, points to help balance the body. Rest, definitely not strenuous activity, is recommended after a hot stone massage, as is rehydration by drinking plenty of water.

Cold stones can be used as an energizer or when there is inflammation in the soft tissue being massaged.

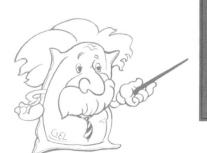

For hot stone massage, the stones should be marble or basalt (lava rock) as these are non-porous and retain heat especially well.

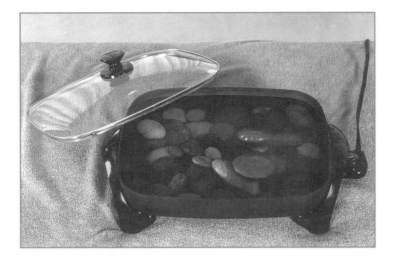

Figure 7.27: The hot stones heater can be a commercial unit or a suitable size electric cooker.

Equipment:

- massage table
- appropriate sheets or towels for draping
- hot stones unit
- tongs
- non-porous stones of various sizes
- oil
- additives (optional)
- chakra crystals (optional)

Procedure:

- Pre-heat the heating unit.
- Have the client lie on the table.
- Undrape the client.

- Remove suitable stones from the water unit with tongs.

- Always ensure the stones are not too hot for the individual.

- Place heated stones or crystals on the appropriate chakra positions (optional). Some therapists place heated stones along the length of the spine at the beginning of the treatment to generate warmth and relaxation. Either type of pre-treatment use helps acclimatize the client to the heat of the stones.

- Pour massage oil into your hands and carefully pick up stones, oiling them as well.

- Perform the massage, turning the stones often to maintain the heat level applied to the tissue.

- Change stones depending on the size of the body part being massaged.

- After every treatment, wash the stones with soap and then boil them for a few minutes. Tea tree oil can be added to the water as a disinfectant.

Figure 7.28: Pre-treatment hot stones placement options.

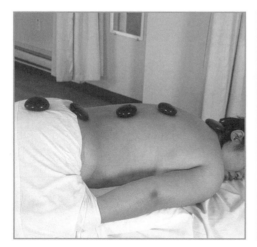

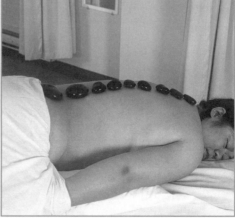

a: Chakra placement.   *b: Spinal row placement.*

Figure 7.29: Hot stone massage.

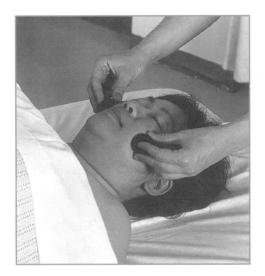

*a: Select smaller stones for
a treatment area like the face.*

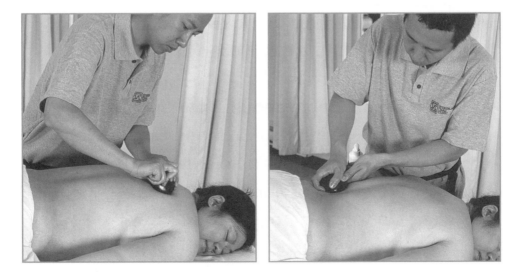

b & c: Hot stone massage of the back.

'Sauna' is the only Finnish word found in the English language. It is believed that there is one sauna for every three citizens of Finland. When in a sauna, Finns have traditionally been swatted with a *vihta*, a bunch of birch twigs that is about 40 cm long. Slapping the skin in the sauna promotes blood circulation and cleanses the skin. People strike the skin not to the point of pain, but just to make the skin tingle. The vihta is used in the summer so the birch boughs are fresh. People should shower or swim after a sauna. Many Finns traditionally cut a hole in the ice of a lake and jumped into the water, or rolled in the snow if there was no lake nearby.

Chapter Eight

Large, Intense Hydrotherapy Treatments

Learning Objectives

After learning the contents of this chapter, the reader should be able to:

- demonstrate an understanding of suitable uses for the treatments

- demonstrate awareness of the intensity level of the treatments and when a client may need a medical opinion

- list the necessary equipment for each application

- explain the appropriate procedure for each treatment

- incorporate these treatments into clinical practice or workplace use as appropriate

- make suitable recommendations for use as home care, or in other locations where a client may have access to the necessary equipment, for example at a spa or fitness club

Russian Jews who moved to the United States developed their own type of bathhouse, called the *shvitz bawd* or *sweat bath* (shvitz = sweat). The *mikhvah* were Jewish ritual baths used for various religious and physical purposes. In the shvitz, cupping was used to relieve many physical ailments; *bahnkes* were glass cups applied to the skin by suction. A rubdown often followed the shvitz. The rubdown was called the *plaitza*, and used soap-covered oak leaves. People would finish up with a steam room or a dip in a pool.

Chapter 8: Large, Intense Hydrotherapy Treatments

The treatments in this chapter involve larger scale, more intense hydrotherapy applications. Some of the treatments mention the option of incorporating additives – additives are discussed in Chapter 9.

Introduction: Large Scale Hydrotherapy Treatments

Large treatments elicit a variety of responses that involve a composite of local, reflex and systemic effects. Factors like full body temperature exposure, water immersion, and steam environments mean that these applications are more intense, have stronger effects than local applications, and are usually more aggressive in therapeutic intent. They are widely used to detoxify the body and improve the skin's ability to eliminate through perspiration. In some cultures saunas, steams or sweats are integral to the concept of physical and spiritual cleansing.

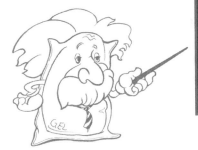

Factors like full body temperature exposure, water immersion, and steam environments mean that these applications are more intense, have stronger effects than local applications, and are usually more aggressive in therapeutic intent.

The intensity of such large scale treatments dictates that they should never be rushed. The time spent in and out of these applications must be kept at a quiet, calm, even pace. Each individual will react differently, so there are no absolutes as to how much time should be spent or what temperatures must be used – consider the information provided in this chapter as guidelines, but modifications to reduce treatment intensity are often appropriate.

In using these treatments in clinical practice and as home care recommendations, it is important to recognize that they are not suitable for everyone. The more intense or aggressive a treatment protocol is, the larger the number of individuals for whom it may be too intense or aggressive. As we have discussed in Chapter 6, there are conditions that contraindicate temperature therapy, especially large scale applications, and those that require substantial adaptation of the chosen treatment. Sometimes medications significantly change physiological reactions to temperature therapies. It is important to recognize such situations, including those that require a medical opinion.

The conditions that most commonly raise concerns related to temperature therapy are:

- cardiovascular conditions

- respiratory conditions

- renal disorders

- diabetes

- pregnancy

- epilepsy

In addition to these, there are numerous other conditions that involve considerations about temperature tolerances, sensory impairment, stages of healing, and so on. There is also the question of where the person's condition falls along the mild-moderate-severe continuum. Mild hypertension, for example, may be fine for many treatments, whereas a moderate case could require substantial treatment adaptation, and a severe or unstable case may contraindicate most temperature therapy applications, especially those covered in this chapter. When in doubt it is important to seek an expert opinion about whether a particular treatment plan is safe or appropriate for the individual case.

General Procedures for Large Scale or Full Body Applications

- Monitor the pulse: The pulse is taken before, during, and after the treatment.

Before treatment:

The client should be at rest. Allow the client to relax first to get an accurate reading; she or he may have rushed to the appointment or feel anxious about the treatment, etc.

During treatment:

The pulse is usually taken every 5 minutes.

During a full body treatment take the carotid pulse because the neck is most easily accessed. The maximum acceptable heart rate increase from the resting pulse is *170 minus the age of the client.*

> The maximum acceptable heart rate increase from the resting pulse is 170 minus the age of the client.

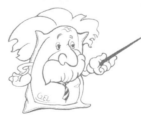

After treatment:

The pulse will usually be slightly higher than the starting rate, but should be lower than during the treatment.

- Monitor the blood pressure, especially with more vulnerable clients or those whose capacity to tolerate the treatment being given is uncertain.

- As discussed in detail in Chapter 5, observe the person closely for signs of discomfort or adverse reactions. Do not leave her or him unattended.

- Replenish cooling elements such as cold neck or forehead compresses frequently during heat treatments.

- Give the client frequent sips of water to avoid dehydration.

- Always remember to have the client dry well afterward so she or he does not become chilled. Cover with a blanket if needed.

- Large scale treatments, especially hot ones, should be followed by a rest period before activity or manual therapy.

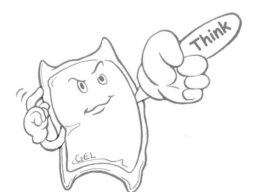

Monitor:
- pulse
- blood pressure
- any signs of discomfort
- adverse reaction indicators

Replenish:
- cold compresses
- water

Steam Treatments

Full body steams use hot water in its gaseous form to increase the core temperature of the body, promoting detoxification by encouraging profuse perspiration. They also promote skin health through increased blood flow to the body surface. Steams are effective at loosening mucus, so are helpful for colds and sinus conditions. Steam treatments are also used to induce physical relaxation, particularly after work-outs, athletics and other types of vigorous exertion.

Caution must be exercised with individuals who have cardiovascular or lung disease – it depends on the severity of the condition but a steam application is frequently too intense. People with diabetes may also need to avoid steams or have the treatment modified because of peripheral vascular impairment. Steam treatments are often inadvisable for pregnant clients because of the increased internal body temperature.

• Sauna

Sauna rooms are built of wood to absorb moisture from the air. This moisture absorption creates a dryer atmosphere than in other types of steams, allowing for easier sweating. Water is poured over heated stones 1-2 times during the treatment to increase the air temperature (or sprayed on electrically heated stones). The most intense heat is found at the top bench level of the sauna. Sitting up also creates a more powerful heat experience, so it is better for the person who is a beginner, is not comfortable with intense heat, or wants to gradually increase the stimulus, to begin lying down or sitting on the bottom levels. A cold compress around the neck also helps moderate the heat.

A sauna is not a rushed affair. The method is to go through repeated periods of heating up, cooling down, and resting (to stabilize the heart rate and blood pressure). As the body heats up, the intensity of the corresponding cold application is increased. By the third heat period, the body is very hot and can possibly withstand a roll in snow or a plunge in a lake. Ideally, the full treatment occurs over 2 hours with a half hour in total actually spent in the sauna.

Equipment:

- towels: one to sit on, one to dry off with, and one for a neck compress (optional)
- buckets, ladle
- drinking water
- loofah to exfoliate the skin (optional)

Procedure:

- Do not rush the treatment; each person goes at her or his own pace.
- Quiet is encouraged.
- Have the person take a cleansing shower and pat dry before entering the sauna.
- Check the person's pulse before the sauna begins and at regular intervals during the treatment.
- Give sips of water throughout the treatment.
- The first heat period lasts 5-15 minutes or until intense sweating begins.
- The next step is a cool/cold shower.
- The shower is followed by a 10 minute rest period.
- Have the client return to the sauna; she or he can sit/lie higher if desired.
- Repeat the process twice, having the person exfoliate with a loofah during the final sauna if desired.
- The final heat period is followed by a final cold shower.
- It is important to complete the treatment with a rest period.

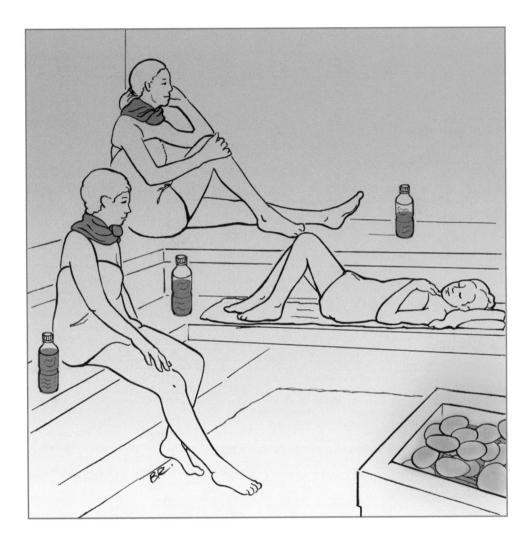

Figure 8.1: In the sauna, it is important to drink water to avoid dehydration. Cold neck compresses can help prevent overheating. Sitting on a lower bench, or lying down, reduces the treatment intensity.

• Steam Cabinet

A steam cabinet is an individual steam treatment unit. It seats one person with her or his head remaining outside the cabinet. Its benefits are similar to those of a sauna, but as an individualized treatment its effects can be more easily controlled and customized.

Equipment:

- steam cabinet
- additives (optional)
- water to fill the steam unit
- towels: to cover the sitting area and the neck opening, for neck or forehead compresses, and for draping and drying the client
- drinking water
- non-glass cup and straw

Procedure:

- Take the client's resting pulse.
- Have the cabinet ready (pre-heated, seat height checked, water level checked).
- Add ingredient(s) to the water if desired.
- Place towels on and over the front of the seat to protect the backs of the legs.
- Have a mat or towel on the floor for the client's feet.
- Assist the person into the cabinet.
- Apply a cold compress to the neck and/or forehead as needed.
- Cover the neck opening with dry towels to prevent leakage of steam.
- Give sips of water every 5-10 minutes or when requested.
- Change the compress(es) when no longer cold, and wipe the face.

- Check the client's carotid pulse since it is accessible.

- Assist the client out after 10-30 minutes, or sooner should the client feel uncomfortable or dizzy. The average treatment time is 20 minutes; 5-10 minutes is stimulating, 15-20 minutes is sedating.

- Give a washing or have the person take a cool/cold shower.

- Post-treatment rest is recommended.

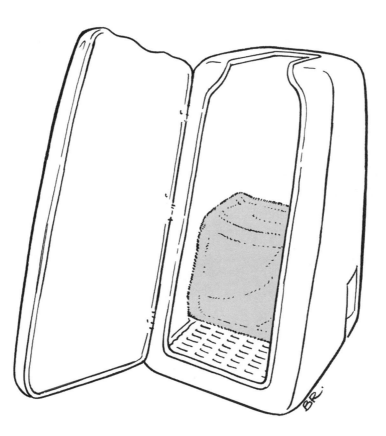

Figure 8.2: When setting up the steam cabinet, use a thick towel to cover the seat and protect the client's legs from the heating unit located under the seat. Place another towel or a mat on the floor for the client's feet.

Figure 8.3: Steam cabinet treatment.

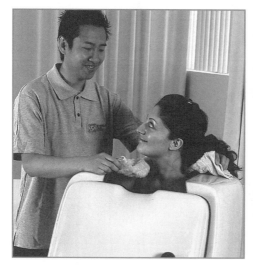

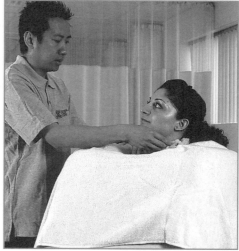

a: Start by seating the client comfortably and applying a cold neck compress.

b: Use a large towel to make a seal between the cabinet opening and the compress.

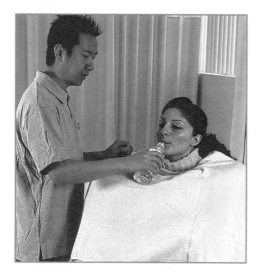

c: Provide sips of water to maintain hydration.

• Facial Steam

A facial steam involves the use of water in gaseous form on the face and upper torso, with the steam being breathed in through the nose and mouth.

Facial steams are useful for easing respiratory congestion by helping to loosen mucus in sinuses, bronchial passages, and lungs. They are often combined with essential oils such as eucalyptus to achieve these effects. They also help facilitate expectoration, especially when combined with tapotement. Facial steams are inappropriate for serious respiratory diseases involving reduced gaseous exchange in the lungs, such as emphysema.

Equipment:

- pot
- large sheet and blanket
- wooden grid (improvise with wooden spoons or something similar, if necessary)
- additives (optional)
- stool and table
- boiling water
- towels (to cover pot; as a compress for back of neck)

Procedure:

- Have the individual disrobe down to the waist to facilitate sweating, then cover her or him with a sheet or towel.
- Have a pot of hot water ready and add any appropriate ingredients.
- It is best to have a grid over the top of the pot: sometimes people feel faint, and the grid prevents any possibility of burning from inadvertent contact with the pot.
- Place a towel over the whole pot: This towel can be rolled back and forth by the client to adjust the intensity of the steam being released.

- It is best if the client is seated on a stool and the pot is placed close in front of the client on a low table.

- Have the client lean over the pot, and drape a large sheet and blanket over the client's head and upper body as well as the pot.

- Have the person stay in the steam for up to 20 minutes, allowing for 'air breaks' if necessary.

- Apply a cold compress to the back of the neck if the client desires, or if there is a history of headaches.

- Wash off the face and torso with cool water and encourage rest.

- Avoid chilling.

- If massaging after, it is good to focus on the sinuses and chest, using vibration, shakings, and tapotement.

Figure 8.4: Preparing the pot.

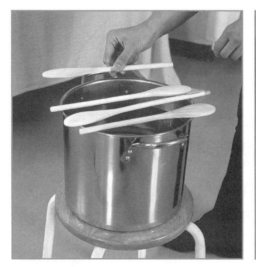 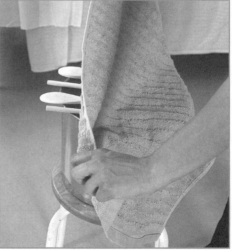

a: For safety, use a wooden grate or spoons.

b: A folded towel allows adjustment of steam intensity.

Figure 8.5: Facial steam treatment.

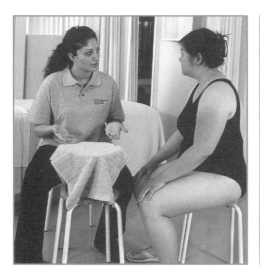

a: Make sure the client understands the treatment.

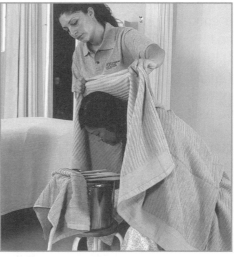

b: With the client's face over the pot, cover with a towel.

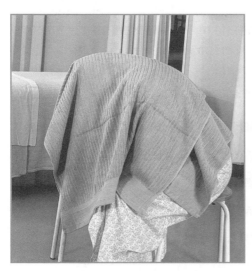

c: The client's upper body is 'tented' over the pot.

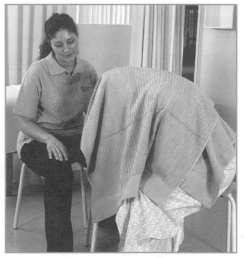

d: Check on the client's comfort regularly.

Baths

In a bath, the entire body is immersed in water except for the head. A bath is good for inducing relaxation, and is an ideal medium for using therapeutic additives. Epsom salts and essential oils are among the many types of substances that can be added to bath water. Additives are discussed in Chapter 9.

• Hot Baths

Hot bath temperatures should be between 36° and 38°C (97°-101°F). Although cooler than the usual heat range, this temperature has the effects of hot when used for a full body immersion. Prolonged submersion in water that is too hot can be debilitating. An exception is the Epsom salts bath, where the temperature can be as high as 39°-44°C (102°-111°F). Careful monitoring of the pulse rate and intake of liquids during hot baths is important, particularly with individuals who are weak, old, or very young, or who have cardiovascular problems. With cardiovascular conditions where use of baths is appropriate, adjustments can be made by modifying the temperature and/or lowering the water level to below the level of the heart, and by allowing the water to drain at the end of the treatment so that pressure on blood vessels normalizes before the person gets out of the tub.

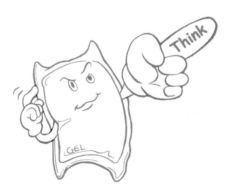

Careful monitoring of the pulse rate and intake of liquids during hot baths is important, particularly with individuals who are weak, old, or very young, or who have cardiovascular problems.

With cardiovascular conditions where use of baths is appropriate, adjustments can be made by modifying the temperature and/or lowering the water level to below the level of the heart, and by allowing the water to drain at the end of the treatment so that pressure on blood vessels normalizes before the person gets out of the tub.

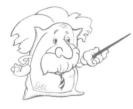

- **Contrast Baths**

Contrast baths are helpful for addressing sluggish circulation, fatigue, lethargy and depression. Large scale contrast baths require careful monitoring, particularly if there are any cardiovascular concerns, because of the increase in vascular activity. The hot application should be 38°-43°C (100°-110°F) and the cold 5°-13°C (40°-55°F).

General Equipment:

- deep bath tub
- contrast baths require two baths or pools
- bath pillow
- towels

General Procedure:

- Prepare the tub(s) with the appropriate temperature water.

- Add any additives.

- For a hot bath, have the person sit in the tub for 15-20 minutes. A cold compress around the neck can be used if needed.

- Hot baths are best followed by a cool/cold wash or shower unless further sweating is required.

- For a contrast bath, the person generally sits in the hot water for 3-5 minutes and in the cold plunge for less than 1 minute – this cycle is repeated twice or more. Variations of this cycle, as outlined in Chapter 4, may be appropriate.

- Be sure the client is dry after the treatment to avoid chilling.

- Rest should generally follow any intense heat treatment.

Figure 8.6: Client care during the bath treatment.

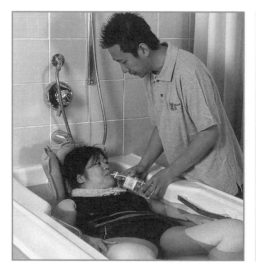 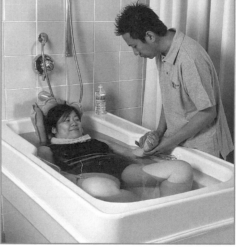

| *a: Ensure comfort and hydration.* | *b: Monitor the radial pulse.* |

Sitz Baths

A sitz bath immerses the body from navel to mid-thigh with the upper body and limbs left out of the water. Sitz baths can be warm/hot, cold, or contrast treatments. They are mainly used to treat the abdominopelvic area including the urinary, reproductive, and lower digestive organs. There is an inexpensive home care version that sits on the toilet seat and is commonly used to treat the perineum after childbirth.

Note: A warm foot bath can be given in conjunction with a hot sitz bath to minimize pelvic congestion.

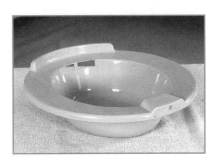

Figure 8.7: Home care perineal sitz bath.

General Equipment:

- sitz bath/large bucket/bathtub
- towels: for compress, if required; for drying off
- large blanket or sheet
- footstool/foot bath

General Procedure:

- The client can keep the upper body clothed to prevent chilling or can be wrapped in a large towel or a blanket.
- Check the resting pulse before the treatment and at intervals as needed for good monitoring.
- Check the water temperature – see Baths above.
- Using a bathtub: the person's legs can be above the water level on a plastic stool in the tub with the arms along the tub rim, or the legs and arms can rest on the edges of the tub or the individual can sit sideways in the tub with the arms out and the legs dangling or on a stool.

- Explain the procedure, particularly the positioning.

- Assist the client into the sitz bath if needed.

- Leave the client in for the time specified – see Baths above.

- The person may need to rest afterward.

• Warm Sitz Baths

Warm sitz baths promote circulation, help to decongest the abdominal viscera, relax muscle tension, and increase circulation to the skin. They are helpful for conditions such as hemorrhoids, dysmenorrhea (painful menstruation), and for postpartum perineal care.

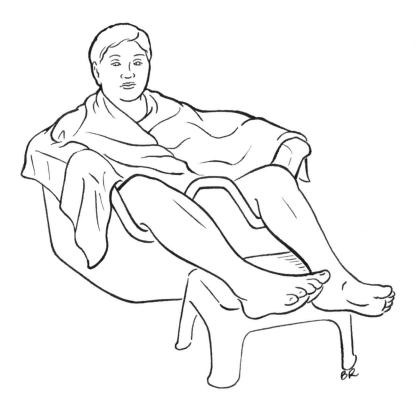

Figure 8.8: Commercial sitz bath.

Equipment:

- warm water at 36°-38°C (97°-100°F)
- Epsom salts or cider vinegar can be added to the bath for detoxification

Procedure:

- Apply a cold compress to the neck if necessary.
- Cover the client's upper body with a sheet/blanket.
- A warm foot bath can be done in conjunction with the sitz bath.
- The treatment lasts approximately 10-20 minutes (shorter duration for a tonic effect; longer for a sedative effect).
- The treatment can be finished with a cool/cold wash by pouring water over the bathed area, or with a quick cool shower.

• Cold Sitz Baths

Cold sitz baths are brief. They are helpful for increasing blood flow into the abdominopelvic contents for conditions such as constipation and hemorrhoids. They are also used for menorrhagia (abnormally heavy menstrual bleeding) and following childbirth. Cold sitz baths should be avoided during active bladder or kidney infections.

Equipment:

- cold water at 12°-21°C (53°-70°F)

Procedure:

- Ensure the client is warm before the treatment begins.
- Cover the upper body with a blanket during the treatment.
- Leave the person in the bath for 10-60 seconds.
- Follow with rest or massage.

Figure 8.9: Sitz bath options in a regular tub.

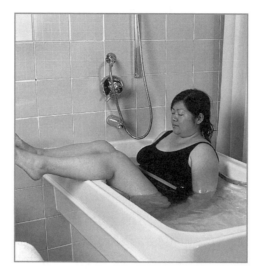

a: Seated sideways.

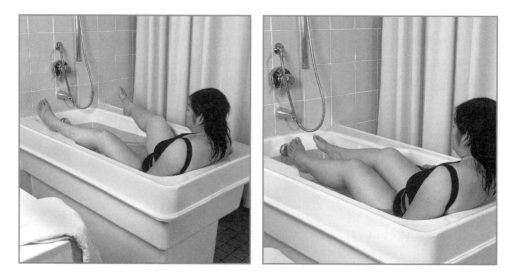

b: Feet on tub rim.   *c: Feet on plastic stool.*

• Contrast Sitz Baths

Contrast sitz baths promote circulation in the abdominopelvic area. They are particularly helpful with constipation, hemorrhoids, and postpartum care. They can be used post-surgically to promote internal healing once the incision is healed and any vaginal bleeding, if present, has stopped.

Equipment:

- 2 sitz baths or big buckets
- water at 36°-38°C (97°-100°F) and 12°-13°C (54°-56°F)
- foot bath (optional)
- sheet and blanket

Procedure:

- If the person is chilled, do a warm foot bath first.
- Assist the client into the tubs each time.
- The duration of the application is warm for 3 minutes, then cold for 30 seconds.
- Repeat the process 3-5 times.
- You may not need to cover the person when she or he is in the cold sitz bath because of its short duration.
- Generally this treatment should be followed by rest.

Whirlpool

A whirlpool uses air or water jets in a tub to agitate warm/hot water against the submerged body part(s). It can be a full body or partial treatment. Whirlpools are helpful for increasing overall circulation. They are commonly used as a sedative to relax the individual and for warming up or soothing tissues before or after stretching, exercise, or massage. Arthritic joints, muscle stiffness, and overall tension can be addressed by a whirlpool treatment.

Whirlpools can also use cold and contrast temperatures, comparable to those given above for sitz baths. Adjustments to the heat:cold ratio can be made (discussed in Chapter 4). Individuals with multiple sclerosis can benefit from cool submersion applications and a whirlpool can be used in milder cases.

The use of whirlpools should be carefully considered for anyone who has cardiovascular conditions, including high or low blood pressure. The temperature may need to be adjusted, the size of the application modified, and for clients with mild/moderate cardiac problems, a suitable treatment may require adjusting the water level to below the heart.

Equipment:

- whirlpool
- drinking water, non-glass cup
- cold water and bucket for compresses
- large towel to drape and dry client; small towel for compress
- bath pillow
- additives (optional)

Procedure:

- Take the client's resting pulse.
- Prefill the tub to the desired level and temperature. This is generally 40°-43°C (104°-109°F), but with cardiac or vascular concerns 32°-35°C (90°-95°F) may be more appropriate.
- Add any ingredients.

- Place the seat in the appropriate position.

- Adjust the jets to the desired height and intensity.

- Assist the client into the whirlpool and position comfortably.

- Place cold compresses around the neck.

- Turn on the jets after the client is in the water.

- The treatment generally lasts 10-25 minutes – this amount of time is relaxing; less time is stimulating.

- Check the pulse regularly.

- Change the compress as needed.

- With hot applications give sips of water frequently.

- After the appropriate time, turn off the jets and assist the client out. For clients with cardiovascular or motor impairments, let the water out of the tub before helping the client out.

- Prepare a cool/cold shower or full body washing.

- Disinfect the tub after each use.

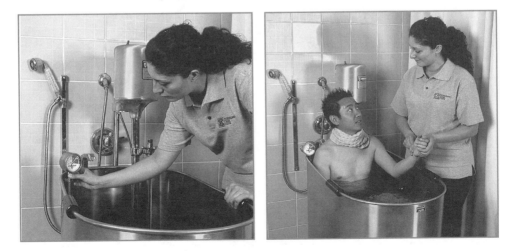

Figure 8.10a & b: With whirlpool treatments, keep a close check on water temperature and client comfort.

Spray

A spray is similar to a shower, but the spray of water is administered by the therapist. Sprays are more aggressive treatments than showers because the therapist fans or jets the water to increase the percussion aspect of the water pressure. The pressure is not as forceful as a high power jet and should not be uncomfortable or painful. Sprays can be full body applications or directed at a specific body part or tissue area. They can be used to help prepare the body for more aggressive treatments, or to improve an individual's tolerance of cryotherapy.

Cold and contrast sprays increase blood flow to the body surface, stimulating the skin. They also act as an overall tonic, increasing energy and alertness. The cold water should be 10°-15°C (50°-60°F). For people who are unused to or dislike cold, the temperature can start at 15°-25°C (60°-80°F) and then be reduced.

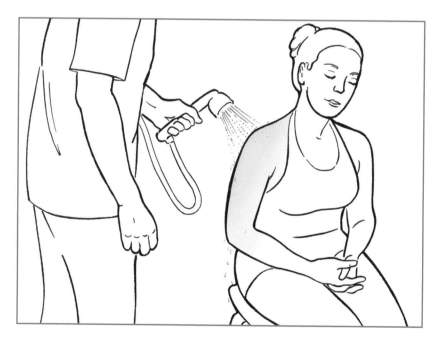

Figure 8.11: Spray treatment.

For contrast sprays you must have two showers, or nozzles with separate temperature controls, or know *exactly* how to go back and forth between the two desired temperatures. The hot component is 36°-38°C (97°-100°F) and the cold is 12°-15°C (54°-59°F).

Tepid and hot sprays are relaxing and help address muscle fatigue. Tepid water is between 25°-33°C (80°-92°F), while hot is 38°-41°C (100°-105°F).

Equipment:

- shower (two for contrast treatments) with a shower head or nozzle in the control of the therapist
- stool, if required
- towels for drying

Procedure:

- Adjust the water to the appropriate temperature.
- Have the client seated or standing depending on which body part is being treated, e.g., seated for the back, standing for legs.
- Spray the water on the target tissue, gradually increasing the flow pressure to the desired volume.
- A cold spray lasts 30 seconds to 3 minutes.
- Tepid sprays last 4-6 minutes.
- Hot spray treatments last between 1 and 6 minutes.
- Contrast spray treatments generally have a heat:cold ratio of 3 minutes hot to 1 minute cold, although this can be modified as discussed in Chapter 4.
- Monitor the client for headache or dizziness, especially with full body applications.

"The cure for anything is salt water – sweat, tears, or the sea."

Isak
Dinesen

Chapter Nine

Additives

Learning Objectives

After learning the contents of this chapter, the reader should be able to:

- explain different methods by which aromatherapy oils can be used

- describe the effects of some commonly used essential oils

- list some conditions with which the use of essential oils is appropriate

- describe how and when to use mustard, ginger, oatmeal and baking soda as temperature therapy additives

- explain some of the key functions of magnesium in the human body

- explain the primary methods by which Epsom salts and apple cider vinegar are used therapeutically

- list some uses for castor oil

- describe how to apply castor oil compresses and castor oil paste

Hippocrates (460-375 B.C), the Greek father of modern medicine, is also the father of *thalassotherapy*, therapy by bathing in sea water. He discovered the reduced risk of infection and the relief of pain after using sea water on wounds. He taught that water could be used both as a tonic and as a sedative.

Chapter 9: Additives

Herbs, salts and plant extracts have been used in baths and other water treatment practices for centuries. Adding a substance to a hydrotherapy application can enhance its effects. In this chapter we will consider common additives that are readily available: essential oils, mustard, Epsom salts, and apple cider vinegar. We will also look briefly at castor oil, which is not technically an additive but is a commonly used temperature therapy substance. In choosing to incorporate any of these substances in clinical practice or home care, it is important that only high quality products be used to ensure their therapeutic value.

Essential Oils

During the Great Plague of the Middle Ages, medical practitioners carried walking sticks with a *cassolette* (perforated container) filled with aromatics. These plant materials acted as personal antiseptics, and would be held up to the nose when visiting any contagious cases. Whether true or not, it has been widely reported that these medical practitioners were virtually immune to the Plague.

Essential oils are the volatile oils distilled from plants. A variety of plant parts, such as the flower, leaves, fruit or roots, can be used for extracting the oil. Essential oils enter the body through the skin and the respiratory tract and can produce a number of different effects. Many also have antiseptic properties. In their pure form they can be very potent and *should always be well diluted when applied to the body*, never neat.

Essential oils can be employed in temperature therapy in a variety of ways. They can be used individually, or two or three oils can be blended together to enhance their therapeutic properties. Baths, inhalations, and compresses are the temperature therapy applications that lend themselves best to using essential oils as additives. In a full body bath, only 5-7 drops are necessary for the oil to have a therapeutic effect. Foot or hand baths require only 2-3 drops. For a shower, the usage is a little different. Run the shower a little hotter than normal to heat up the bathtub and create steam. After the water has run for a couple of minutes, reduce the heat, cover the drain, and put 7 or 8 drops of the essential oil(s) into the shower stream as the water descends. Enter the shower and inhale deeply for several minutes, then allow the water to drain. Alternatively, this procedure can be done at the end of the shower.

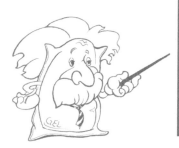

Essential oils are the volatile oils distilled from plants. They enter the body through the skin and the respiratory tract and can produce a number of different effects. Baths, inhalations, and compresses are the temperature therapy applications that lend themselves best to using essential oils as additives.

For an inhalation, 2-3 drops of an essential oil can be put on a tissue and inhaled during a treatment. For a more aggressive inhalation, the oil(s) can be coupled with steam. Bring 2 cups of water to a boil, allow it to cool slightly, then add 2-5 drops of oil. Have the person inhale the vapours for 5-10 minutes. Putting a towel over the individual's head envelops the steam and increases the concentration of the oil.

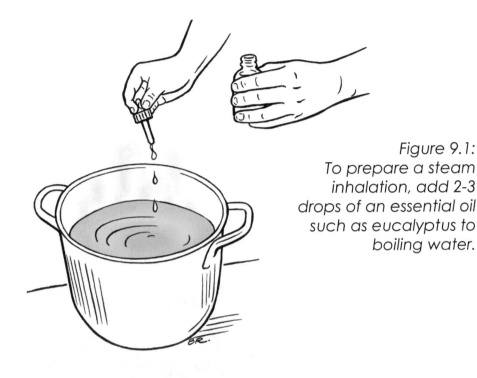

Figure 9.1:
To prepare a steam inhalation, add 2-3 drops of an essential oil such as eucalyptus to boiling water.

To prepare a compress, mix ½ litre (2 cups) of water and 5-7 drops of essential oil. The water can be hot or cold depending on the purpose of the treatment. Soak a piece of linen or cotton in the mixture, wring it out, and place it on the target area. Remove when the hot compress is cooled or the cold compress is heated to body temperature.

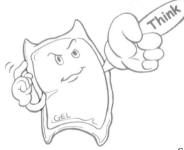

Essential oils can have powerful effects, so it is important to be cautious when using or recommending them. Unless you are trained as an aromatherapist, you should avoid utilizing these oils in more complex prescriptions or case scenarios. When in doubt, err on the side of caution and refer the client for more expert advice. Without additional expertise, practitioners should avoid using essential oils altogether if the individual is undergoing chemotherapy, is pregnant, has high or low blood pressure, or experiences epileptic seizures.

It is also important to realize that, regardless of the general usage of an oil, scents will have individual emotional effects – aromatherapy must be chosen for the person receiving the treatment. For instance, clary sage is a commonly used oil for mood elevation, but if the person doesn't like the smell of clary sage it will not have a soothing effect. Similarly, an oil could have a negative association. A former client once told me she didn't like the smell of lemongrass because it reminded her of lemon-scented cleaning products and therefore housework. People can also have atypical physical reactions to essential oils.

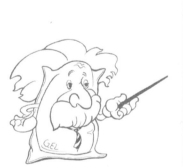

It is important to realize that, regardless of the general usage of an oil, scents will have individual physical and emotional effects.

There is a list of commonly used essential oils in the box below. Peppermint, rosemary, tea tree, and the citrus oils (orange, lemon, lemongrass, lime, grapefruit, etc.) are all refreshing and stimulating oils. Tea tree is a wonderful antifungal oil. Eucalyptus is invigorating and is also an effective decongestant and expectorant that is widely used to relieve cold symptoms. Black pepper, cinnamon, and ginger are examples of warming oils, which are helpful for joint and muscle aches. Clary sage, as mentioned above, is widely used for depression. Lavender is a special oil, as it can be blended with most other oils and works to enhance their qualities. On its own, lavender is calming, as is chamomile. Ylang-ylang and sandalwood are also soothing oils, but they have pungent aromas and can cause headaches if overused. Two very good oils for female concerns, such as menstrual cramps and premenstrual syndrome, are rose and geranium. True rose essential oil is very expensive; geranium is a more affordable substitute.

common essential oils and their effects

oil	effect
black pepper	warming
chamomile	soothing
cinnamon	warming
citrus oils	refreshing, stimulating
clary sage	mood elevating
eucalyptus	invigorating, decongestant
geranium	female hormone balancing
ginger	warming
lavender	calming; enhancing other oils' effects
peppermint	refreshing, stimulating
rose	female hormone balancing
rosemary	refreshing, stimulating
sandalwood	sedating
tea tree	stimulating, anti-fungal
ylang-ylang	soothing

Epsom Salts

Epsom salts is a preparation of magnesium sulphate, named in the 18th century for the town of Epsom in southern England where the salts were originally obtained from a local mineral spring.

Epsom salts is widely used to ease stress, reduce headaches, improve sleep, decrease muscle tension and soreness, and detoxify the body. A large functional component of Epsom salts is magnesium, an element that is vital to many of the body's physiological functions.

Modern farming methods do not emphasize crop rotation, a practice that helps maintain mineral balance in the soil. As a result, the foods we eat often contain less magnesium than is required for optimal body health.

Magnesium helps regulate electrolyte levels and is necessary for good cardiovascular and nervous system function. Its role in calcium regulation is not well publicized but magnesium is vital in skeletal and heart muscle contraction and in healthy blood clotting. It also plays a role in stress management and mental health, since it is important in the production and maintenance of serotonin (a neurochemical involved in balancing moods).

Diffusion through the skin is often a more efficient method for magnesium absorption (www.epsomsaltcouncil.org) because some foods and medications inhibit optimal assimilation of magnesium through the digestive tract. Epsom salts baths, then, are a good option for increasing the body's magnesium level.

Epsom salts can be used in a variety of temperature therapy applications. For a compress, mix 250 ml (1 cup) of Epsom salts with 2 litres (½ gallon)

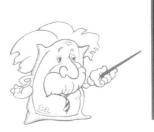

> **Diffusion through the skin is often a more efficient method for magnesium absorption because some foods and medications inhibit optimal assimilation of magnesium through the digestive tract.**

of warm water and place on or wrap around the sore area. Add 250 ml (1 cup) of Epsom salts to a foot bath or 500 ml (2 cups) to a hot full body bath, and soak for 15-20 minutes to help detoxify and soothe. The person should shower or rinse off afterward. Epsom salts baths are often recommended following exercise or manual treatments like massage therapy.

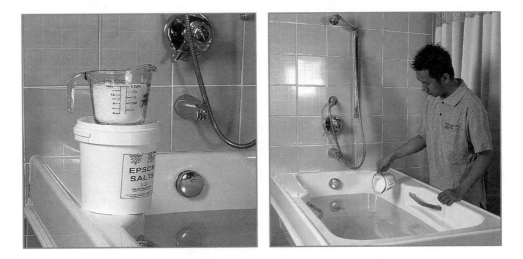

Figure 9.2a & b: The classic Epsom salts application is a hot bath, to which is added 2 cups of Epsom salts.

Apple Cider Vinegar

Apple cider vinegar is another popular additive. It detoxifies, purifies, promotes digestion, and decreases arthritic pain. Instead of using Epsom salts, use 250-500 ml (1-2 cups) of apple cider vinegar in a warm tub. It can also be added to heating compresses, hot towel rolls and fomentations.

Ginger

Ginger is a warming substance that can be applied by using its essential oil, or its root grated fresh or in dried powder form. Ginger water is widely used to address the symptoms of colds and bronchitis through increasing sweating and reducing phlegm production. It also helps to increase circulation and detoxify the body, and is used to address pain, stiffness and cramps. Ginger also decreases injury healing time and helps to boost the immune system.

To make ginger water you will need a large heat-maintaining pot – an enamelled pot is ideal. Have ginger powder (or grated ginger), small cotton towels, a large thick towel, and a cotton or cheese cloth bag available. Boil

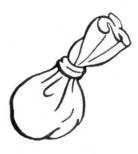

about 4 litres (1 gallon) of water. Place 15 ml (1 tbsp) of ginger for every litre of water into the cotton bag or cheese cloth. Tie it closed snugly but not so tightly that water cannot run through the ginger. After the water boils, reduce it to a simmer and place the ginger bag into the water. It should simmer for about 5 minutes – do not let the water re-boil once the ginger has been added.

For the easy creation of a compress, take a small towel and fold it into thirds lengthwise, placing the middle in the hot ginger water and leaving the ends dry so it can be easily wrung out. Once you have done so, refold the towel to the desired width to fit the target tissue. Apply to the skin, being careful that it is not too hot. Cover with the large, dry towel to maintain the heat, and replace the compress as needed. The compress will likely need to be replaced every 3-4 minutes to maintain therapeutic warmth. The entire treatment should take 20-30 minutes. Expect the skin to become very reddened, or to darken substantially depending on the skin colour of the individual.

Ginger water is only very potent for about 2-3 hours, but can be used for up to 24 hours. Instead of throwing out the remaining water, you can add it to a bath or a footbath.

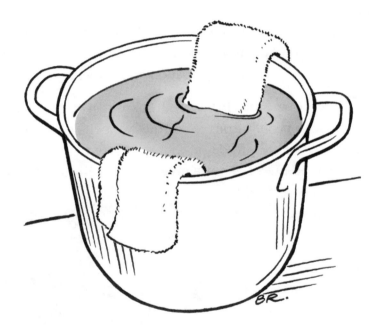

Figure 9.3: It is easier to wring out the hot ginger water compress if you leave some of the towel dry at each end.

Mustard

> The ancient Greeks believed that mustard was created by Asklepios, the god of healing, as a gift to humankind.

Mustard is widely used in poultices or foot baths to treat cold symptoms. For a poultice for an adult, mix 45 ml (3 tablespoons) of flour with 15 ml (1 tbsp) of dry mustard and add enough water to create a paste. Apply to the target tissue and cover, being sure to keep the area moist. For children, change the recipe to 5 ml (1 teaspoon) soda, 5 ml (1 tsp) dry mustard, and 5 ml (1 tsp) flour. Avoid using this application on very young children.

Some people experience skin irritation from direct contact with the mustard paste and may benefit from an alternative method of preparation: place the mustard mixture inside a thin cloth (e.g., a dish towel). This application can be placed in a microwave for pre-heating if desired. Position the compress on the target tissue and leave on for 15-30 minutes.

For use in a foot bath, add 15-45 ml (1-3 tbsp) of mustard flour (3:1 flour to mustard proportion) in a deep foot bath and soak for 10-15 minutes. For a full body bath, mix 125-250 ml (½ to 1 cup) with cold water to make a paste. Press the mixture through a cloth into warm bath water and soak in the bath for 10-15 minutes.

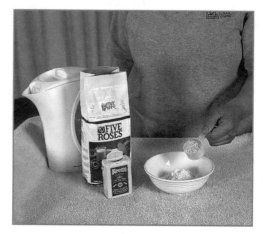

Figure 9.4:
Mustard paste preparation.

Figure 9.5: Mustard poultice treatment.

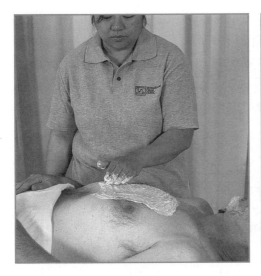

a: *Spread a layer of mustard paste on the target tissue.*

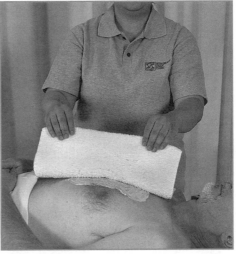

b: *Cover immediately with a small dry towel.*

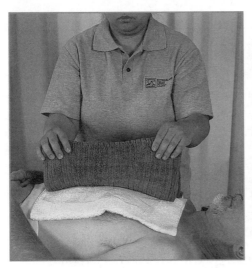

c: *Add a hot compress (optional).*

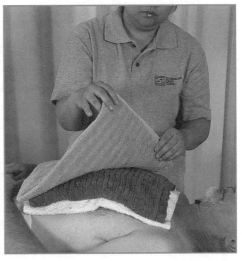

d: *Cover the application with a thin dry towel.*

Baking Soda

Baking soda, also known as sodium bicarbonate or bicarbonate of sodium, is found in mineral deposits throughout the world. Baking soda is a common household product with many uses related to cleaning, deodorizing, beautifying, and cooking. It is also used in baths and as a paste to address a number of conditions, especially ones that involve skin itch such as insect bites and hives.

In addition to itchy skin conditions, baking soda baths and pastes can help relieve sunburn, fever, foot fatigue and foot odour, cold sores, acne, and rough skin. A strong baking soda solution also helps to clean a wound and decrease local swelling around a lesion.

To prepare a baking soda paste, add water to an adequate amount of baking soda to make a thick paste. Apply it directly to the affected tissue area. For baths, use 2 cups of baking soda in a full body bath and 45 ml (3 tablespoons) in a foot bath.

Oatmeal

Oatmeal is used as a mild exfoliator to soften the skin, and to provide relief from itchy skin conditions. It is also reported to soothe and improve diaper rash when used in a baby's bath.

To employ oatmeal therapeutically, use a muslin bag of about 5 cm x 5 cm (2" x 2"), either purchased or sewn. The bag is filled with raw oatmeal, leaving enough room for expansion of the oatmeal when wet. Tie the bag closed with string or an elastic band. Hold it under the bath water stream as the tub is filling so the oatmeal can soften the water. The person then soaks in the tub for 20-30 minutes, using the bag as a scrubber to provide mild exfoliation if desired.

Castor Oil

> The first documented use of castor oil is from about 1550 B.C., in *Ebers' Papyrus*, which is one of the oldest preserved medical documents.

Castor oil, also known as Palma Christi ('the hand of Christ'), has been used in healing for centuries. Taken orally as recommended by practitioners such as naturopaths, castor oil is used for general detoxification, increasing lymphatic drainage, and decreasing the burden on the kidneys. It is also employed in compress form to address gall bladder concerns, constipation, headaches, menstrual cramps, arthritic pain, and skin disorders.

As a paste, castor oil can effectively address such concerns as calluses and ingrown toenails. Take ½ ml (1/8 tsp) of baking soda and mix with 3-4 drops of castor oil in your palm, then massage the mixture into the target tissue. For a longer treatment, wrap a towel around the tissue and leave for several hours.

A heated castor oil compress is particularly helpful as part of a treatment protocol to reduce the visibility and restriction of scars. 75-125 ml (5-8 tablespoons) of castor oil absorbed into 3 or 4 layers of a natural fibre are placed on the target area, covered with plastic, and overlaid with heat. For home care it may be more convenient for the person to warm a castor oil infused cotton facecloth or small towel in the microwave – it should be warmer than skin temperature but not hot. The compress can be kept on for ½ to1 hour, or as long as overnight. If used in a clinical setting as a preliminary to friction therapy, 10-15 minutes will suffice. The home care poultice can be re-used if stored in the freezer. Castor oil will stain, so an old T-shirt or towel should be recommended to cover the compress. (As a tip, soda water works well for cleaning up castor oil spills.)

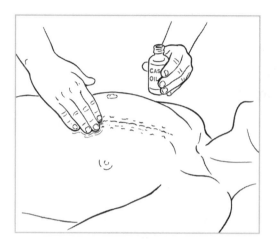

Figure 9.6:
A heated castor oil
compress is particularly
helpful as part of a
treatment protocol to
reduce the visibility and
restriction of scars.

Figure 9.7: Heated castor oil compress.

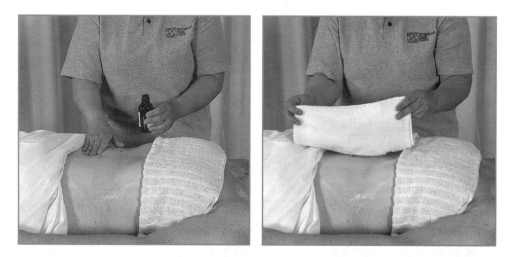

a: Apply the castor oil
liberally to the skin surface.

b: Place a thin towel over
the oil (optional).

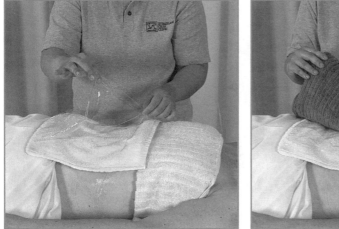

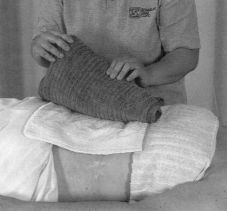

c: Apply a thin sheet of plastic wrap.

d: Place a hot compress on top of the application.

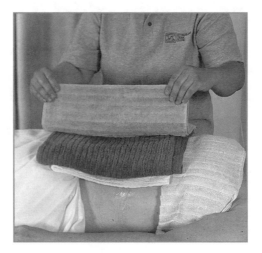

e: Cover with a small dry towel.

In the next chapter, we will complement the temperature therapy and additives information covered in recent chapters with a discussion of recommending temperature therapy as home care.

*Dr. Vincent Preissnitz
(1799-1851) of Silesia
(part of what is now
Germany) mangled his
hand and healed it with
cold compresses. He
was a strong advocate
of the healing powers
of water.*

Chapter Ten

Home Care Temperature Therapy

Learning Objectives

After learning the contents of this chapter, the reader should be able to:

- use lay language to make a temperature therapy recommendation for home care

- recommend appropriate home care treatments that are suitable to the client and use readily available items

- advise clients what to notice and what to report back about their home care applications

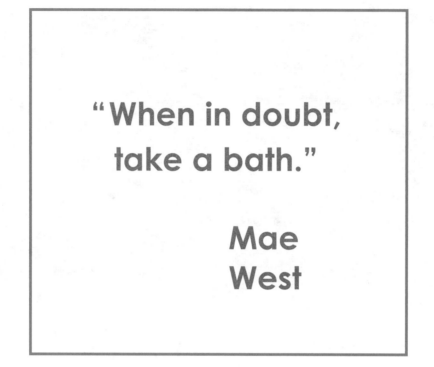

"When in doubt,
take a bath."

Mae
West

Chapter 10: Home Care Temperature Therapy

Home care is a very important part of most treatment plans. One of the benefits of temperature therapy is that it lends itself readily to home use applications. People can enhance their comfort and their healing processes by incorporating home treatment recommendations from their therapists into their daily routines.

Client Education

As therapists we must educate our clients about the appropriate uses of heat and cold and provide them with accessible, affordable suggestions about how to perform their own treatments at home. When they consistently do the home care component of their treatment plans, clients see faster, better results. We can also give them a good general understanding of how to make self-treatment decisions in everyday life.

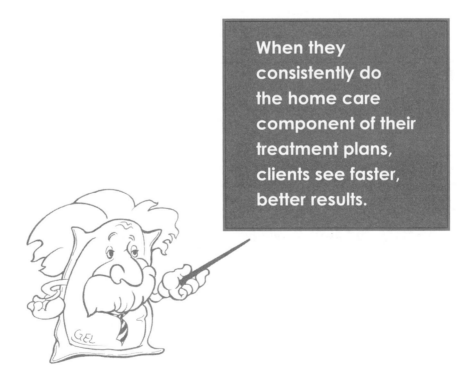

When they consistently do the home care component of their treatment plans, clients see faster, better results.

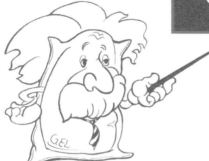

> **While a cold treatment will rarely aggravate a condition, heat most certainly can.**

The most common concern about home use of temperature therapies is people's inclination to always choose heat. Heat tends to feel comforting, while cold usually does not. However, while a cold treatment will rarely aggravate a condition, heat most certainly can. For instance, if applied to a recent injury that is sore and swollen, heat will intensify the inflammatory process and make the pain and swelling worse. *It is often the case that it is better to use nothing than to use heat.* It is essential, then, to explain the risks and benefits of temperature therapy use at home in an easily understandable way. Education about the beneficial uses of cold is often quite eye-opening for the lay person.

Most clients do not have a strong background in human physiology. It is therefore important to describe what temperature agent to use, and why, in clear and simple language. Discussing 'retrostasis' or 'vasoconstriction' is not suitable with most people – unless you are both up for a lengthy explanation – and will keep them from gaining the knowledge they need in order to understand the treatments and their effects. The terms that relate to temperature therapy can usually be simplified for easy accessibility.

common temperature therapy terms in everyday language

technical term	becomes...
thermotherapy	heat treatment
cryotherapy	cold treatment
core temperature	inner temperature of the body
shell temperature	skin surface temperature
vasodilation	widening (opening) of blood vessels
vasoconstriction	narrowing of blood vessels
derivation	movement of blood toward the location of the heat application
retrostasis	movement of blood from the skin surface deeper into the body's organs
hyperemia	redness that occurs when a lot of blood moves into a tissue

Recommending Home Treatments

When recommending a home care regimen, the first thing to do is to make sure that it is clear what is being treated. If the chief concern is pain, what is the cause? Some pain is better treated with cold, some with heat. The best compliance occurs when the client understands what the temperature treatment is designed to address.

Explain *how* the application will help address your mutually agreed goals. Remember to use understandable language based on the individual's level of knowledge. A simple explanation will suffice, for example, "Your sprained ankle is inflamed, causing swelling around the injury and into your foot. Adding heat will just increase the inflammation, so you need to use cold. The cold will help to reduce your pain, and will narrow the blood vessels to bring the swelling down." Or, "Because of the way you sit at work, your neck and shoulder muscles have tightened up in this tense position. When muscles are tight for long periods of time, they don't get the blood supply they need to work properly, and they become sore. Heat on your shoulders will encourage the muscles' blood vessels to open and bring in more blood." Double check that the person understands the explanation you have given.

Because not all home care will be an exact reproduction of temperature therapy done in the therapist's clinic, it is essential to describe (and sometimes demonstrate) the recommended treatment thoroughly and plainly. The type of heat or cold source, the specific temperature, the duration and frequency of treatments, the time of day, and the use of any coupling agents need to be explained. As with a clinical treatment, include appropriate post-treatment activities in your recommendation.

As an example of what can happen with poorly understood instructions, here is an anecdote from a colleague: a client was instructed to do contrast bathing at home by another health professional who was treating his hand injury. What he did as contrast bathing was 30 minutes of hot followed by 10 minutes of cold, after which his hand was incredibly swollen! It is

It is a good idea to have brief, clearly written hand-outs describing home care treatments you recommend routinely.

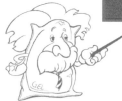

not difficult to see how this might have happened with an instruction that was too quickly given. It is often a good idea to have brief, clearly written hand-outs describing home care treatments you recommend routinely.

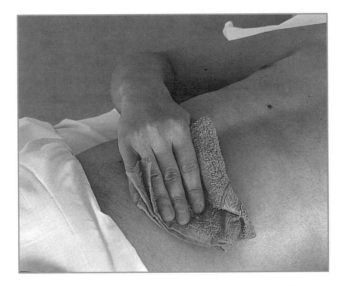

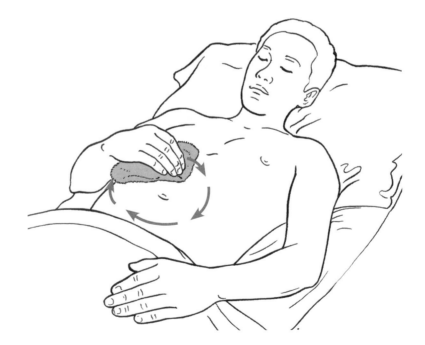

Figure 10.1: A self-administered cold abdominal washing before sleep can help address insomnia or constipation.

Many people do not have 'proper' temperature therapy tools, and will not take the time to set up complex or time-consuming treatments, so your suggested applications need to incorporate straightforward purchases or be modified to what is in the home. You should also be prepared to make suggestions about where to purchase items like Epsom salts or paraffin wax preparations.

Gel packs are now readily available in a variety of sizes in common retail outlets, so they are excellent home temperature therapy tools. If the person has a few hot/cold gel packs, magic bags, or temperature beanbags, these can be used for most purposes. Wherever possible, accommodate to the heating and cooling agent(s) that the person will commit to using, and be realistic given where on the body the application must go. What follows are some additional examples of easy, inexpensive options, most of which are applied wrapped or covered by a thin hand towel or dish towel.

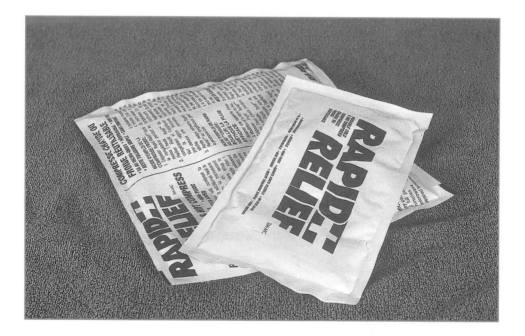

Figure 10.2: Gel packs are readily accessible, easily used, and come in several shapes and sizes.

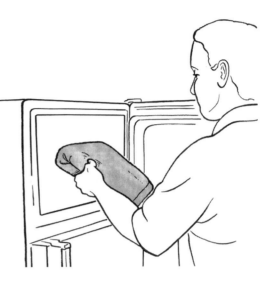

Figure 10.3:
Frozen towels are very
inexpensive and easy
to prepare at home.

For cold applications:

- plastic bag filled with popcorn (unpopped) kept in the freezer

- bag of frozen vegetables such as peas

- frozen juice tin (a good fit for some surfaces, e.g., palmar surfaces of hands or for rolling under feet)

- frozen towels

- ice cubes in a plastic bag

For heat applications:

- hot water bottle

- wet towels heated in a microwave

- castor oil on a cotton facecloth warmed in the microwave (especially good for scars, contractures, tight iliotibial bands)

For contrast applications:

- examples from the hot and cold lists above used in combination

- double sinks can be filled with different temperature water for hand or arm baths

Be sure to make the recommended treatments realistic for the individual's lifestyle and schedule in order to increase the opportunity for compliance. Advising the average person to rub ice on a sore knee for 15 minutes every 3 hours is probably unrealistic. Recommending applying a cold pack for a minimum of 10 minutes while the individual eats daily meals, watches an evening television program, and reads before going to sleep will sound much more practical and achievable. Remember to include the person in the process of determining a suitable home treatment plan. As they see good results, people often become willing to try more complex types of home care applications.

Finally, advise the individual about how the skin should look and feel during and after the treatment. Discuss common symptoms of negative reactions and what to do if one occurs. Review the treatment plan with the person at each appointment, particularly when she or he is just starting home temperature therapy.

> **Ask the person to note any changes resulting from the temperature therapy and to tell you about them at your next session. When you regularly request information about home care treatments and consider it with due seriousness, you gain a more rounded view of the case.**

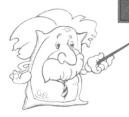

Monitoring Outcomes

Make sure you have a method for evaluating the results of the home treatment plan. Did the pain and swelling in her ankle lessen? Did the muscle soreness ease in his neck? Ask the person to note any changes resulting from the temperature therapy and to tell you about them at your next session. When you regularly request information about home care treatments and consider it with due seriousness, you gain a more rounded view of the case. This dialogue also helps emphasize the importance of the client's role and encourages compliance. As with applications you would do as a therapist, if there are no improvements, make changes in the treatment plan.

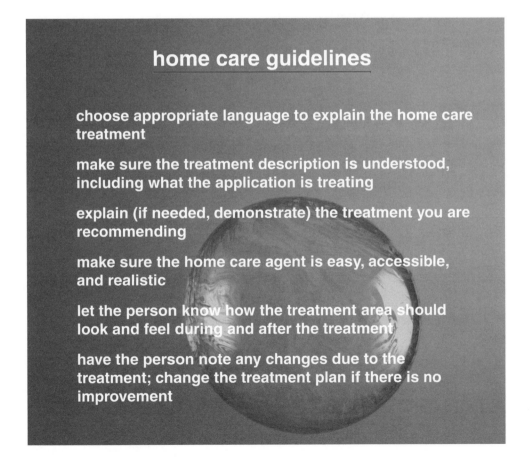

home care guidelines

choose appropriate language to explain the home care treatment

make sure the treatment description is understood, including what the application is treating

explain (if needed, demonstrate) the treatment you are recommending

make sure the home care agent is easy, accessible, and realistic

let the person know how the treatment area should look and feel during and after the treatment

have the person note any changes due to the treatment; change the treatment plan if there is no improvement

The earliest known Mayan community sweat house is believed to date back to 900 B.C. in Belize. The Mayan sweat houses' purposes are thought to have been threefold: physical cleansing, bodily purging, and spiritual preparation.

Appendix

celsius/fahrenheit conversion

It is important to be able convert Celsius to Fahrenheit and vice versa. There are formulas for changing one temperature system to the other.

- To convert Celsius to Fahrenheit, the formula is [x(1.8)+32], where x = °C. Every 1°C is about 1.8°F.

- To convert Fahrenheit to Celsius, the formula is (x-32)(0.56), where x = °F. Every 5°C is about 9°F.

conversion table

°C	°F		°C	°F	
-273	-459	*(absolute zero)*	41	105.8	
-40	-40		42	107.6	
-5	23		43	109.4	
0	32	*(water freezes)*	44	111.2	
5	41		45	113	
10	50		50	122	
15	59		55	131	
20	68		60	140	
25	77		65	149	
30	86		70	158	
35	95		75	167	
36	96.8		80	176	
37	98.6		85	185	
38	100.4		90	194	
39	102.2		95	203	
40	104		100	212	*(water boils)*

temperature range chart

The temperatures used in cryotherapy and thermotherapy vary depending on the types of applications being administered. The following examples demonstrate the ranges of cold and heat that we use commonly in temperature therapy treatments.

	temperature range	application examples
very cold	-5° to 0°C (23°-32°F)	ice cubes, ice bags
cold	1°-10°C (33°-50°F)	cold gel pack
	4°-27°C (40°-80°F)	bath: limbs: 4°-15°C (40°-60°F) body: 18°-27°C (65°-80°F)
warm	36°-44°C (50°-80°F)	bath: hand: 36°-44°C (98°-111°F) limbs: 37°-40°C (98°-104°F) body: 37°-39°C (98°-102°F)
hot	52°-57°C (125°-135°F)	paraffin wax
	74°-77°C (165°-170°F)	hot pack
contrast bath	total range 5°-42°C (40°-107°F) cold 5°-15°C (40°- 60°F) hot 40°-42°C (104°-107°F)	

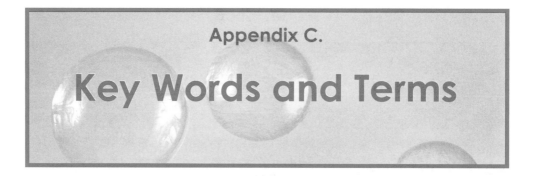

Appendix C.
Key Words and Terms

- **Activities of Daily Living (ADL)**
everyday activities and routines in the client's life; a useful reference for the temperature therapist to help determine her or his tolerance of hot and cold modalities

- **Additives**
substances of various types that can be added to temperature therapy applications to enhance their effects

- **Anaesthetic Effect**
numbing effect, or relief of pain

- **Analgesic Effect (Analgesia)**
painkilling effect

- **Arterial Trunk Reflex**
increase or decrease of blood flow through an arterial trunk will produce the same effect in its smaller distal branches

- **Cardiac Output**
the amount of blood pumped out of the heart each minute, a factor of heart rate and venous return volume

- **Caution**
an element in an individual's case that causes the therapist to be more cautious and observant when using temperature therapy and to implement treatment adaptations suited to the case

- **Contracture**
results when connective tissue conforms to a continuously held position; collagen fibre cross-linkages create a stiffer and less pliable fascial structure

- **Contraindication**

a condition, disease, or other element in an individual's case that prevents the use of some or all types of temperature therapy

- **Contrast Temperature Therapy**

the use of alternating applications of hot and cold temperature therapy in order to create a cycle of vasodilation and vasoconstriction to 'flush' the tissues

- **Core Temperature**

the temperature of the body's internal structures; 37°C (98.6°F) is the norm for the human body

- **Coupling Agent/Medium**

a medium or material used with a temperature therapy agent to increase or modify the treatment effects

- **Cryoagent**

a type or form of cold application

- **Cryotherapy**

the therapeutic use of cold applications

- **Dehydrated/Dehydration**

a drop in the body's fluid content below optimally required levels

- **Depressive Reaction/Effect**

when a response to a stimulus involves slowing, reducing or suppressing tissue activities

- **Derivation**

drawing of fluid, in this context blood, from its main pathway toward a tissue area with a lower blood volume; active derivation requires expenditure of energy and passive derivation does not

- **Detoxify/Detoxification**

promoting the removal or elimination of toxic elements and waste products from the body, though increasing filtering activity in organs of elimination such as the liver and kidneys and/or via increased perspiration

- **Dyspnea**

a primary symptom of respiratory disorders, meaning shortness of breath or breathing difficulty; can be exacerbated by steam environments or intense heat

- **Edema**

extra accumulation of fluid in the interstitium (spaces between cells); often called swelling

- **Essential Oil**

a volatile oil distilled from a plant; can be used therapeutically to achieve specific effects

- **Exfoliator**

a physical stimulus that removes the top layer of dead cells from the skin

- **Frostbite**

damage to the skin and underlying tissues from excessive cold

- **Frostnip**

initial indication of excessive cold in a tissue, manifesting as paleness, numbness and/or tingling of the skin; first stage in the development of frostbite

- **Home Care**

the adaptation of various therapeutic modalities, including temperature therapy, for home use as part of a treatment plan

- **Homeostasis**

the results of numerous inter-related physiological activities that keep the body's systems and processes operating within healthy parameters

- **Hunting Response**

cyclic vasodilation and vasoconstriction that occurs in issue that has been cooled below 10°C (50°F)

- **Hydrostatic Pressure**

the pressure a fluid exerts in all direction on the walls of its container, for example, blood on blood vessel walls

- **Hydrotherapy**

the use of water in any of its three forms (liquid, solid, gas) as a temperature medium to achieve therapeutic effects

- **Hyperemia**

the tissue is holding a higher than usual volume of blood; in the skin and subcutaneous tissue this results in visible redness

- Hypothalamus

the part of the brain that plays the central role in thermoregulation; it receives temperature information from the body tissues and monitors the temperature of its own blood flow and initiates heat-conserving and heat-losing activities as needed to maintain homeostasis

- Hypoxia

inadequate oxygen supply for a tissue's needs; leads to damage, especially if sustained

- Inflammatory Response

the body's general response to injury and other types of tissue disruption; the response is geared to support immune defense, protect the site and prepare for repair, and moves through acute, sub-acute and chronic stages

- Insulator (insulation)

a substance, like fat, that conducts temperature poorly and consequently can prevent heat or cold from entering or leaving a tissue area

- Ischemia

delivery of oxygenated arterial blood to a tissue is less than its current need

- Local Effect

an effect that is created in the specific tissue area to which a stimulus like temperature therapy is applied

- Metabolism

the cumulative result of chemical processes and activities occurring in a body tissue, system, or the body as a whole

- Muscle Guarding

protective muscle contraction in the vicinity of an injury or a site of pain

- Muscle Spindle Reflex

a reflex that responds to stretch on a muscle by protectively increasing the muscle's contraction level; the muscle spindle is the embedded stretch receptor that monitors stretch on the muscle belly

- Negative Reaction

a response to a temperature therapy treatment that is unexpected and undesirable

- **Patch Testing**

applying a sample version of a proposed temperature therapy application to a small area of the target tissue to evaluate the response

- **Poultice**

an application that is a variation of a compress, in which a moist paste, often heated, is applied to the target tissue using towel or other fabric as a coupling medium; also called a plaster

- **Reflex Effect**

an effect that is created when the nervous system mediates a tissue response to a stimulus, for example, when a temperature therapy application applied on the body surface produces a response in a muscle or organ because of nervous signals transmitted as a result of the stimulus

- **Retrostasis**

fluid is being mobilized from the body surface into organs and other deeper structures

- **Sedative Effect**

a calming, soothing or relaxing effect; can also be synonymous with Depressive Effect

- **Shell Temperature**

the temperature of the body's surface structures, which is typically 1-6°C less than the core temperature

- **Specific Heat**

the capacity of a substance to hold or store heat

- **Stimulating Effect**

when a response to a stimulus involves activating, increasing, or speeding up tissue activities

- **Strengthening Reactions**

stressors such as temperature therapy, as long as they are applied within healthy parameters, stimulate the body to improve its capacity to tolerate or withstand the stressor

- **Systemic Effect**

an effect that is produced broadly in a body system or in the whole body

- **Temperature Therapy**

utilization of a range of temperature applications to achieve therapeutic effects

- **Thermal Conductivity**

the capacity of a substance to transfer or conduct heat to another substance

- **Thermoagent**

a type or form of heat application

- **Thermoregulation**

the body's system for maintaining its temperature within normal healthy parameters; includes heat losing and heat conserving activities

- **Thermotherapy**

the therapeutic use of heat applications

- **Tonic Application**

treatments, often incorporating cold or friction or both, that are used to stimulate a strengthening reaction, making the body more resilient

- **Treatment Intensity**

the range and strength of an application's effects, resulting from such factors as temperature differential between the application and the body, size of application, temperatures used, speed and duration of application, and so on

- **Vascular Flush**

the primary effect of contrast temperature therapy, which creates alternating derivation and retrostasis (vasodilation and vasoconstriction) that mobilizes blood through the treated tissue and enhances delivery of nutrients and removal of wastes; also called circulatory whip

- **Vasoconstriction**

contraction of smooth muscle in a blood vessel wall resulting in narrowing of its internal passageway; this decreases the volume of blood permitted to flow through it

- **Vasodilation**

relaxation of smooth muscle in a blood vessel wall resulting in expansion of its internal passageway; this increases the volume of blood able to flow through it

- **Viscous/Viscosity**

the lower the fluid content of a substance such as blood, the more viscous, or thick, it is; the more fluidity in the substance, the lower its viscosity

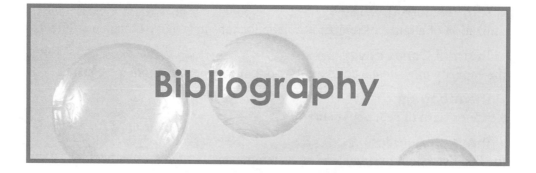

Bibliography

American Cancer Society. (n.d.). Retrieved February 27, 2006, from http://www.cancer.org/docroot/MBC/content/MBC_2_3x_Radiation_Therapy.asp?sitearea=MBC

A Modern Herbal. (n.d.). Retrieved January 14, 2006, from http://botanical.com/site/column_poudhia/articles/__11914.html

Anderson, K., Anderson, L. & Glanze, W. (Eds.). (1998). *Mosby's Medical, Nursing & Allied Health Dictionary* (5th ed.). Toronto: Mosby

Associated Bodywork & Massage Professionals. (n.d.). Retrieved January 16, 2006, from http://www.massagetherapycentre.com/epsomsalt.html

Austrian Cultural Information System of the Federal Ministry for Education, Science and Culture. (n.d.). Retrieved February 27, 2006, from http://www.aeiou.at

Bélanger, A-Y. (2002). *Evidence-Based Guide to Therapeutic Physical Agents*. Baltimore: Lippincott, Williams & Wilkins

Boyle, W. & Saine, A. (1988). *Lectures in Naturopathic Hydrotherapy.* Sandy, OR: Eclectic Medical Publications

Cankars. (n.d.). Retrieved January 16, 2006, from http://www.cankar.org=http://www.visitfinland.com/w5/index.nsf/(pages)/Secrets_of_the_Sauna?OpenDocument&np=A

Centre for Disease Control and Prevention. (n.d.) Retrieved January 30, 2006, from http://www.bt.cdc.gov/disasters/winter/guide.asp#health_emergencies

Circle of Life Holistic Programs. (n.d.). Retrieved January 14, 2006, from http://www.circle-of-life.net/colonicdetails.html

Cyber Bohemia. (n.d.). Retrieved January 17, 2006, from http://www.cyberbohemia.com/Pages/sweat.htm

Dr. Emily Kane, ND. (n.d.). Retrieved January 16, 2006, from http://www.dremilykane.com

Driftwood Handmade Wooden Baths. (n.d.). Retrieved February 27, 2006, from http://www.driftwood.ie/woods.html

Epsom Salt Council. (n.d.). Retrieved January 16, 2006, from http://www.epsomsaltcouncil.org/about_news_bureau.htm

Fowlie, L. (2003). *An Introduction to Aromatherapy: course notes.* Unpublished manuscript.

Get a Life/The Principles of Detoxification. (n.d.). Retrieved January 30, 2006, from http://www.getalife.net.au/cancer/packs_html

Global Health Solutions. (n.d.). Retrieved January 30, 2006, from http://www.watercure.com

Health Enotes. (n.d.). Retrieved February 27, 2006, from http://www.health.enotes.com

Healthy Concept Online. (n.d.). Retrieved January 14, 2006, from http://www.healthyconcept.ca/cellwater.html

Internet Health Library. (n.d.). Retrieved January 30, 2006, from http://www.internethealthlibrary.com/Therapies/Hydrotherapy.htm#top

Light Network. (n.d.). Retrieved January 15, 2006, from http://home.claranet. nl/users/lightnet/health/messages/ginger.html

Marieb, E. (2004). *Human Anatomy & Physiology* (6th ed.). San Francisco: Pearson Benjamin Cummings

Michlovitz, S. (1996). *Thermal Agents in Rehabilitation* (3rd ed.). Philadelphia: F.A. Davis Co.

Minnesota Public Radio. (n.d.). Retrieved January 30, 2006, from http://www. news.minnesota.publicradio.org

Natural Family Online. (n.d.). Retrieved January 16, 2006, from http://www. natural-family.com/3nut-64-magnesium.htm

Nikola, R. (1998). *Creatures of Water: Hydrotherapy Textbook.* Salt Lake City: Europa Therapeutic

Old Newark Web Group. (n.d.). Retrieved January 16, 2006, from http:// newarkmemories.com/memories/583.php

O'Rourke, M. (1995). *Hydrotherapy & Heliotherapy: Natural Healing with Water, Herbs & Sunlight.* Miami: Educating Hands Inc.

Orthopedic Technology Review. (n.d.). Retrieved January 16, 2006, from http://www.orthopedictechreview.com/issues/julaug02/pg18.htm

Oxford Aromatherapy. (n.d.). Retrieved January 30, 2006, from http://www. oxford-consultants.tripod.com/Index.htm

Persad, R. (2001). *Massage Therapy & Medications.* Toronto: Curties-Overzet Publications Inc.

Planet Herbs. (n.d.). Retrieved January 16, 2006, from http://www. planetherbs.com/courses/sample_lesson.php

Psych Symposium. (n.d.). Retrieved February 26, 2006, from http://
psychsymposium.com/categorylist_html?cat_id=1

Resourceful and Ingenious Uses of Baking Soda. (n.d.). Retrieved January 30,
2006, from http://www.bakingsodabook.co.uk/health-tips-using-baking-soda.
shtml

Salt Works. (n.d.). Retrieved February 27, 2006, from http://www.saltworks.
us/salt_info/si_WaterTherapy.asp

Scandinavica. (n.d.). Retrieved January 15, 2006, from http://www.
scandinavica.com/culture/tradition/sauna.htm

Shankar, K. & Randall, K. (2002) *Therapeutic Physical Modalities*.
Philadelphia: Hanley & Belfus Inc.

The Soy Daily. (n.d.). Retrieved January 14, 2006, from http://www.
thesoydailyclub.com/SFC/adventist02.asp

The World's Healthiest Foods. (n.d.). Retrieved January 14, 2006, from http://
www.whfoods.com/genpage.php?tname=nutrient&dbid=75#nutrientdescr

Tortora, G. & Grabowski, S. (2003). *Principles of Anatomy & Physiology*
(10th ed.). Hoboken, NJ: John Wiley & Sons.

Victorian Turkish Baths. (n.d.). Retrieved January 15, 2006, from http://www.
victorianturkishbath.org/1INTRODUCTION/INTRODUCTION.htm

World Wide School. (n.d.). Retrieved January 16, 2006, from http://www.
worldwideschool.org/about.html

Index

thrombus, 142, 143, 157
thyroid gland, 21
tonic applications, 188, 242, 283
tonic friction applications, 188–97
       cold mitten friction, 189–91
       dry brushing, 192–95
       salt glow, 196–97
towels
       alternating, 173–75
       contrast, 178
       frozen, 271
       hot, 173
       hot towel roll, 176–77
transient ischemic attack (TIA), 158
treatment area (of body), 108–9
treatment guidelines, 116–22
treatment intensity, 283
treatment priorities, 99
treatment room and equipment, 117
Turkish baths, 88

ulcerative colitis, 153
unable to communicate, 147
unreliable feedback, 147

varicose veins, 158–59, 207
vascular disorders, peripheral, 84, 104, 149, 151, 155
vascular flush, 89, 283
vasoconstriction, 15–16, 20, 22–23, 37–38, 55, 267, 283
vasodilation, 15–16, 21–23, 30, 267, 283
       contralateral, 78
       derivation, 38, 64–65
       during inflammation, 47
       and permeability, 39, 40, 41
vasomotor effects, 32
vasomotor impairment, 157, 159
venous blood, 47, 48
venous negative reactions, 125–26, 129

vertigo, 154
vinegar, apple cider, 254
visceral reflex referral zones, 31
visceromotor effects, 32
viscosity, 283

warm therapies. *See* heat and
  thermotherapy
warm *vs.* hot, 63
washings, 198–201
        abdominal, 201, 269
water, properties of, 24–25
West, Mae, 262
whirlpool, 240–41
wounds, 59, 189, 196